America's New Slavery?

FMRI Technology!

Functional Magnetic Resonance Imaging!

Or America's Salvation?

All Americans Should Be Concerned!

America's New Slavery?

FMRI Technology!

Functional Magnetic Resonance Imaging!

Or America's Salvation?

All Americans Should Be Concerned!

Jose Collazo

Library of Congress Control Number:		2010904588
ISBN:	Hardcover	978-1-4500-7378-3
	Softcover	978-1-4500-7377-6
	Ebook	978-1-4500-7379-0

This book was printed in the United States of America.

To order additional copies of this book, contact:
Xlibris Corporation
1-888-795-4274
www.Xlibris.com
Orders@Xlibris.com
75947

CONTENTS

To my Lord and God, whose guidance, love, and strength have given me the courage to finish this book!

To my mother, sister, grandparents, aunts, uncles, and cousins, who have all given me a little something to enrich my life!

To all those people who stood behind me, beside me and protected me, may God bless you and bring you to his glory!

INTRODUCTION

For over thirteen-plus years, I have been trying to prove that the U.S. government has the ability to read a person's thoughts. Functional magnetic resonance imaging is one name for this technology. I now have absolute proof that such technology exists. Now it is up to American citizens to ask, how has this technology has been used? Why was it not used to stop Bin Laden? How is it being used?

If you check YouTube, search *mind reading*, and look for a *60 Minutes* broadcast from January 4, 2009, by Leslie Stahl on FMRI technology, you will find more insight. If you check YouTube for *Conspiracy Theory* by Jesse Ventura on truTV on the HAARP program, you will find more insight.

I have made many Freedom of Information Act requests to the CIA, NSA, NRO, etc., and have gotten interesting responses. Sometimes they do not respond, sometimes they refuse to respond, sometimes they misplace my paperwork—very interesting responses over the years. I requested information on technology that read the thoughts and patterns of the human brain, among other requests. I presented lies, obstruction-of-justice claims, and my new proof to several courts; and no one orders a hearing or a discovery. I have four present cases in the Eastern District Court in Central Islip, New York: *Roman v. NSA* (no. 09-2947), *Roman v. NRO* (no. 09-2504), *Roman v. CIA* (no. 09-3344), and *Roman v. NSA et.al.* (no. 09-4281). If half of the documents I requested from these agencies are released, we will have much more proof.

The real question is going to be, Was the technology used for good; or was it used to promote someone's evil agenda? We, the people, must question these things, and may God have mercy on those who violated our constitution and civil liberties. It is because of President Nixon and Watergate, Iran-Contra Affair, the forty-four-plus politicians, rabbis, arrested in New York and New Jersey in 2009 for money laundering and bribery that we must check. It is because of the evil, corrupt men in the world that we must have a system of checks and balances. Please read my papers of support and come to your own conclusion.

Today, February 15, 2010, new evidence has been found that really alarms me. In the September 2001, volume 49-5 bulletin of the United States Department of Justice Executive Office for United States Attorneys Office of Legal Education, Washington, D.C. 20535. "Forensic Evidence", page 38. Future improvements, the most promising avenues for deception detection include the work with FMRI technology. You will find a copy of this introduction. This technology can be used to do evil or good.

America's salvation could be in these technologies' hands. For those who believe in God and the final judgment. Who has already used this technology?

1. The criminal justice system?
2. On politicians?
3. In business?
4. Anybody who could afford it?

Forensic Evidence

In This Issue

September 2001
Volume 49
Number 5

United States
Department of Justice
Executive Office for
United States Attorneys
Office of Legal Education
Washington, DC
20535

Kenneth L. Wainstein
Director

Contributors' opinions and
statements should not be
considered an endorsement
by EOUSA for any policy,
program, or service

The United States Attorneys'
Bulletin is published pursuant
to 28 CFR § 0.22(b)

The United States Attorneys'
Bulletin is published bi-
monthly by the Executive
Office for United States
Attorneys, Office of Legal
Education, 1620 Pendleton
Street, Columbia, South
Carolina 29201. Periodical
postage paid at Washington,
D.C. Postmaster: Send
address changes to Editor,
United States Attorneys'
Bulletin, Office of Legal
Education, 1620 Pendleton
Street, Columbia, South
Carolina 29201

Managing Editor
Jim Donovan

Assistant Editor
Nancy Bowman

Law Clerk
Brian Burke

Internet Address
www.usdoj.gov/usao/
eousa/foia/foiamanuals.html

Send article submissions to
Managing Editor, United
States Attorneys' Bulletin,
National Advocacy Center
Office of Legal Education
1620 Pendleton Street
Columbia, SC 29201

b. Sensors

Polygraphy can also benefit from a fresh look at its sensors and source of information. Advancements in sensor technology are not well reflected in the configuration of current polygraphs, which have fallen behind other technologies in the physiological fields of study. Not only are more sensitive and comfortable sensors needed, there are many sensors as yet unexploited. Among the candidates for new measures are pupilometry, skin potential, thermography, pulse transit time, and impedance cardiography.

c. Signal Analysis

The government has underwritten developmental projects for automated analyses of polygraph data. The government-funded polygraph algorithm, and other commercially produced analytical tools, have performed well in cross validations. The principal use, and most successful application, of automated algorithms have been in single-issue polygraph testing. Accuracy of the algorithms with confirmed cases is about 90%, making them very useful in the field.

X. Future Improvements

The act of deceiving begins as a cognitive event in which the deceiver decides to communicate information to mislead someone. The cognitive process has neural underpinnings, but the neurological mechanisms involved in deception are not well understood. Central Nervous System or brain research is the next logical advance for the detection of deception. While most existing psychophysiological detection of deception methods, such as the polygraph, have looked for indicators well downstream from the cognitive event of deception, emerging technologies offer promise in identifying deception at its cortical source.

The most promising avenues for deception detection include the work with functional magnetic resonance imaging

(fMRI), High Definition event-related potentials (HD-ERP) and Thermal Image Analysis. All three methods use patterns of activity to infer specific processes. Each uses advanced technology and automated analysis, and provides a unique perspective on mental processes. Spatial information, such as the location of activity within the brain, can be derived from images produced by the fMRI. If a brain location is uniquely implicated in the act of deception, the fMRI is a logical tool to determine whether that location has been activated. The presence or absence of activation in that specific region of the brain could be used as a deception indicator. However, this method requires very large and expensive equipment, restricting its deployability to the field. For this reason, scientists do not see fMRI as the first choice in new technology for detecting deception in the immediate future.

High Definition Evoked Response Potential (HD-ERP) uses scalp sensors to detect electrical signals from the brain. Already, the equipment is potentially portable, and could be developed into a turnkey system. It is one of the most promising new approaches on the horizon. ERPs, in contrast to fMRI, have already been used to detect guilty knowledge. Guilty knowledge tests, however, have very limited utility in the field. As a criterion for usefulness, a brain wave device must be capable of identifying deception with a high validity, a goal for current DoDPI-funded university research.

Thermal Image Analysis (TIA), the detection of patterns of heat from the skin, is a strong candidate technology. The application of TIA to the detection of deception may offer a non-invasive method for determining the veracity, or at least the emotional state, on an individual. With a parallel approach, Dr. Paul Ekman has shown that concealed emotions are revealed through "leakage" in facial expression, called microexpressions. The leakage is unconscious, and careful attention to it might be used to detect deception. Dr. Jeffrey Cohn has automated the analysis of facial expression. The marriage of TIA and Dr. Eckman's theory may prove extremely beneficial to the development of this future sensor. Future research may also find this technology useful to augment other technical deception detection methods.

What awaits America and the world—a new wild, wild West in our minds and privacy. All I know is that all should be concerned, and investigations and guidelines must be in place.

On the next two pages, you will find some of my first real evidence that such a technology really exists. One is by *Technology Review*, explaining FMRI technology; the other, an outline on the *60 Minutes* broadcast on mind reading and FMRI technology.

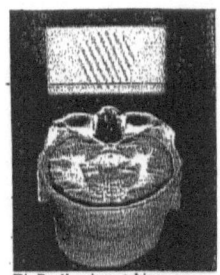

Big Brother is watching you: Researchers used fMRI to peer into the visual cortex of a subject and accurately predict which of two images (circular grating, above) he was holding in his short-term memory. The experimenters used specialized algorithms to tease out subtle patterns in brain activity (represented here in red and green) specific to that image in order to make the call.
Credit: Stephanie Harrison and Frank Tong

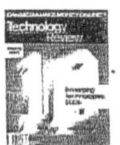
Functional magnetic resonance imaging (fMRI) looks more and more like a window into the mind. In a study published online today in   , researchers at   report that from fMRI data alone, they could distinguish which of two images subjects were holding in their memory—even several seconds after the images were removed. The study also pinpointed, for the first time, where in the brain visual working memory is maintained.

Visual working memory allows us to briefly store and act upon specific details from images that we've seen: what color they are, how they're oriented, and how frequently they appear. But how and where these details are stored has remained a mystery. Early visual areas, which are the first to receive and process visual information, don't seem to stay active long enough to do the job. And higher visual areas don't have the machinery to retain such fine-grained details.

"It's been elusive," says   , a neuroscientist at the Bernstein Center for Computational Neuroscience, in Berlin. "This is a truly brilliant study that now convincingly demonstrates that the information about fine-grained contents of visual experience is held online in the early visual cortex across memory periods."

In the study, subjects were briefly shown two subsequent images of a grating, each image oriented at a different angle. They were then given a cue telling them which one to remember. To ensure that the memory was maintained, subjects were shown a third grating several seconds later and prompted to indicate how it was rotated compared with the remembered one. Throughout the whole process, an fMRI scanner monitored activity in four different early visual areas of the brain.

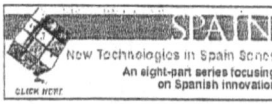

The TR35: Call for Nominations

By analyzing the activity in those areas during the 11-second remembering period, the experimenters were able to determine, with more than 80 percent accuracy, which grating orientation the subject had in mind. To do so, they used a sophisticated analytical tool called a pattern classifier, calibrated for each individual subject by a number of training trials. Rather than simply measuring the overall level of activity, the pattern classifier could probe for patterns in how that activity was distributed across the brain.

This approach turned out to be crucial. Previous studies had unsuccessfully tried to predict subjects' memories by looking at overall brain activity in the early visual areas—an approach that was similarly unsuccessful here. In roughly half of the subjects, overall activity returned to baseline levels soon after the images were removed from view, and in all subjects activity was drastically reduced, making it impossible to decode which image the subject was remembering. But by teasing out specific activity patterns, the pattern classifier was able to reveal the previously hidden information encoded in those areas.

60 Minutes - Mind Reading

De: **Montas, Maria** (MontasM@cbsnews.com)
Enviado: miércoles, 17 de junio de 2009 01:06:38 p.m.
Para: rosalba38@msn.com
       Datos adjuntos:
       image001.jpg (5.0 KB)

Hello Mr. Roman, Please find below cost estimate for the footage you requested. Once you complete the payment form and return to us, we will process your request. Thank you, Maria Montas, CBS News Archives

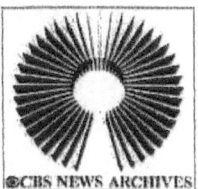

©CBS NEWS ARCHIVES

Date: June 17, 2009
To: Gilbert Roman
E-Mail:

From: **Maria Montas**
          CBS News Information Resources
          524 West 57th Street
          (510/2106)
          New York, NY 10019
Phone: **212-975-6495**
Fax: **212-975-7394**
E-Mail: **montasm@cbsnews.com**

Dear Mr. Roman:

You expressed interest to purchase a DVD of the CBS 60 Minutes segment title "Mind Reading" as reported by Leslie Stahl Jan. 4, 2009 for personal use. We can have the material transferred to a DVD for you, and the costs are as follows:

Footage transfer to DVD: **$ 24.95**
Shipping & Handling: **$ 12.00**
(Plus sales tax)

The DVD will be for **PERSONAL VIEWING USE ONLY. No duplication, excerpting or distribution rights are given. Full payment is required before the material**

DEFENSE ADVANCE RESEARCH PROJECTS AGENCY (DARPA) EXHIBIT

In this section, you will find one of the main players manufacturing FMRI technology and my attempts to see how it is being used. Is it being used by the CIA, NSA, NRO, and FBI in America? God only knows all the answers, and they will answer for any wrong done to Americans in America one day soon. Oh yes, now it is five FOIA cases, *Roman v. DARPA* (no. 09-5633). DARPA refused to answer any FOIA request, and I started an FOIA case against them. The U.S. attorney's office has stated that DARPA is going to release or look for some of my request. I asked for the date FMRI technology was perfected, the report on the first person it was used against, and a present list on all agencies using FMRI technology.

Search Results: fmri

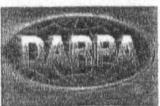

Defense Advance Research Projects Agency
3701 N. Fairfax Ar
Arlington, VA 22203
703-526-6630

SEARCH

SearchResults 1 - 8 of about 11 for fmri . Search took 0.34 seconds.
Sort by date / Sort by relevance

[PDF] INFORMATION PAPER
... Another researcher used functional Magnetic Resonance Imaging (**fMRI**) to image the
brain of human subjects while performing a standard memory task. ...
www.darpa.mil/Docs/PSD_info_paper_Oct07_200807180945043.pdf - 2008-08-20

[PDF] DoD FY 2009 Budget Estimates February 2008
... Determined the functional Magnetic Resonance Imaging (**fMRI**) signatures associated
with expert status on DoD relevant tasks, which include skills that can ...
www.darpa.mil/Docs/DARPAPB09February2008.pdf
[More results from www.darpa.mil/Docs]

[PDF] LCDR Dylan Schmorrow, Ph.D Information Processing Technical Office
... possible have, in large part, been due to the affordability and use of tools such
as functional magnetic resonance imaging (**fMRI**) and electroencephalography ...
www.darpa.mil/DARPATech2002/presentations/ipto_pdf/speeches/SCHMORRO.pdf - 2002-10-29

[PDF] No Slide Title
... Page 5. Distribution Statement A. Approved for public release; distribution is
unlimited. Decade of the Brain **fMRI** Cognitive Revolution Moore's Law Page 6. ...
www.darpa.mil/DARPATech2002/presentations/ipto_pdf/slides/schmorrowIPTO.pdf - 2004-02-25

Defense Sciences Office
... invasive sensors to assess brain states including, but not limited to, EEG
(electroencephalography), MEG (magnetoencephalography), **fMRI** (functional magnetic ...

www.darpa.mil/dso/solicitations/baa06-19mod8.htm - 2009-06-08

Defense Sciences Office
... developed Phase I or Phase II MRI systems for non-invasive, non-structural or
functional imaging of the brain (ie, functional MRI, or **fMRI**; Magnetic Resonance ...

www.darpa.mil/dso/solicitations/baa07-21mod1.html - 2009-06-08

[PDF] "SBIR Successes: Small businesses bridging gaps" Good Afternoon,
... focus on cortical tissue through the skull, and can detect moment-to-moment changes
in the oxygenation of brain regions - similar to those detected by **fMRI**. ...
www.darpa.mil/DARPATech2004/pdf/scripts/SchmorrowScript.pdf

[PDF] Learning and Reasoning: The True Heart of the Mind
... Through **FMRI** and brain imaging techniques, we now have a much clearer idea of how
the brain works than we did in the 1960s and 70s, when most of the current ...
www.darpa.mil/DARPATech2005/presentations/ipto/gunning.pdf - 2005-08-31

In order to show you the most relevant results, we have omitted some entries very similar to the 8 already displayed.
If you like, you can repeat the search with the omitted results included.

DEFENSE SCIENCES OFFICE

HOME	PROGRAMS (A-Z)	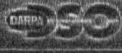	NEWS & EVENTS	SEARCH
STRATEGIC THRUSTS	PERSONNEL	SOLICITATIONS	WORKING WITH DSO	SITE UPDATES

Home > Strategic Thrusts > Training and Human Effectiveness >

Font Size

Neurotechnology for Intelligence Analysts

Program Manager: Dr. Amy Kruse

THRUST AREA

Training and Human Effectiveness

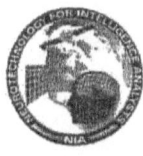

The vision for the Neurotechnology for Intelligence Analysts (NIA) Program is to revolutionize the way that analysts handle intelligence imagery, increasing both the throughput of imagery to the analyst and overall accuracy of the assessments. Current computer-based target detection capabilities cannot process vast volumes of imagery with the speed, flexibility, and precision of the human visual system. Investigations of visual neuroscience mechanisms have indicated that the human brain is capable of responding to visually salient objects significantly faster than an individual's visual-motor, transformation-based (i.e., movement) response.

The NIA Program seeks to identify robust brain signals that are amenable to recording in an operational environment and process these in real time to select images worthy of further review. The program aims ultimately to apply these triage methods to static, broad-area, and video imagery. Successful development of a neurobiologically based image triage system will increase the speed and accuracy of image analysis in a context where the number of acquired images is expected to rise significantly. In sum, the results of the NIA Program will enable image analysts to train more effectively and process imagery with greater speed and precision.

RDT&E BUDGET ITEM JUSTIFICATION SHEET (R-2 Exhibit)	DATE February 2008
APPROPRIATION/BUDGET ACTIVITY RDT&E, Defense-wide BA1 Basic Research	R-1 ITEM NOMENCLATURE Defense Research Sciences PE 0601101E, Project BLS-01

(U) Program Plans:

FY 2007 Accomplishments:
- Demonstrated neurally stimulated tactile feedback by a non-human primate in a reaching and grasping task.
- Developed new methods to discern motor intention in non-human primates.
- Determined the functional Magnetic Resonance Imaging (FMRI) signatures associated with expert status on DoD relevant tasks, which include skills that can make a direct translation to military benefit such as language acquisition, marksmanship, and threat detection.
- Commenced investigations into the neutral basis of expert performance using advanced functional neuroimaging technologies, state of the art spatio-temporal measurement techniques and novel signal processing methods.

FY 2008 Plans:
- Create an interface capable of enabling performance of a complex motor/sensor task through an assistive device.
- Map dynamic functional motor and sensory networks, develop methods for characterizing brain-wide sensor/motor tasks, and determine task performance changes resulting from learning and plasticity.
- Identify the specific brain networks and regions involved in the generation of expert performance; track and classify progression from novice to expert level using functional neuroimaging techniques.

- Investigate non-invasive interventions to increase the speed of expertise development and dramatically accelerate the transition from novice to expert in key military tasks including neuropshyiologically-driven training regimens, neurally optimized stimuli, and stimulatory/modulatory interventions.

FY 2009 Plans:
- Develop prototype training systems to implement the acceleration methodologies for improved training.
- Explore the extrapolation of task specific acceleration techniques from limited domains to wider, more general training applications.
- Identify memory neural codes that are specific to critical work related tasks, enabling possible memory restoration in a brain-wounded warfighter.
- Leverage recent advances in neuroscience and mathematics to construct an integrated mathematical model of the brain that is consistent and predictive, rather than merely biological inspired.
- Develop a theory that overcomes the difficulties present in traditional approaches, such as artificial intelligence and artificial neural network, to properly mode complex human brain processes such as logical reasoning, language, mental computation, and context-dependent mental set.

DEFENSE SCIENCES OFFICE

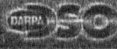

| HOME | PROGRAMS (A-Z) | DARPA DSO | NEWS & EVENTS | SEARCH |
| STRATEGIC THRUSTS | PERSONNEL | SOLICITATIONS | WORKING WITH DSO | SITE UPDATES |

Home > Solicitations >Closed Solicitations >   Font Size 🔲 🔲

Defense Sciences Research and Technology

*Due to the possibility of transcription errors, the official FedBizOpps announcement
takes precedence over this transcription in any disagreement between the two. The
transcription is provided for your convenience only.*

QUICK LINKS

BAA07-21, Part II
02/14/2007

Modification 1
10/19/2007

Modification 2
11/20/2007

General Information

ADDENDUMS

Addendum 1
2/14/2007

Document Type:	Presolicitation Notice
Solicitation Number:	BAA07-21
Posted Date:	Feb 14, 2007
Original Response Date:	Feb 14, 2008
Current Response Date:	Feb 14, 2008
Original Archive Date:	Feb 29, 2008
Current Archive Date:	Feb 29, 2008
Classification Code:	A -- Research & Development
Naics Code:	541710 -- Research and Development in the Physical, Engineering, and Life Sciences

Addendum 2
3/23/2007

Addendum 3
03/27/2007

Addendum 4
4/3/2007

Addendum 5
07/02/2007

Addendum 6
09/13/2007

Addendum 7
10/25/2007

Addendum 8
11/28/2007

Contracting Office Address

Other Defense Agencies, Defense Advanced Research Projects Agency,
Contracts Management Office, 3701 North Fairfax Drive, Arlington, VA,
22203-1714, UNITED STATES

Description

DEFENSE SCIENCES RESEARCH AND TECHNOLOGY PART I
SOL: BAA07-21
DUE: 2/14/08
POC: Ms. Barbara K. McQuiston, DARPA/DSO
FAX: (571) 218-4553
WEB: http://www.darpa.mil/dso/solicitations/solicit.htm
E-MAIL: BAA07-21@darpa.mil

PLEASE SEE ATTACHMENT 1, PART II, BEFORE SUBMITTING TO
BAA07-21

PROGRAM OBJECTIVES, SCOPE AND FUNDING

The mission of the Defense Advanced Research Projects Agency's
(DARPA) Defense Sciences Office (DSO) is to identify and pursue high-

RDT&E BUDGET ITEM JUSTIFICATION SHEET (R-2 Exhibit)	DATE February 2008
APPROPRIATION/BUDGET ACTIVITY RDT&E, Defense-wide BA1 Basic Research	R-1 ITEM NOMENCLATURE Defense Research Sciences PE 0601101E, Project BLS-01

- Deduce how object representation in the mammalian inferotemperal cortex is computed from downstream visual system (V4) inputs using tools from topology, geometry, and statistics.
- Design enzymes with catalytic activity 10x improved from 2007 designs.
- Design proteins with 10x binding affinity to a second target protein.
- Demonstrate autonomous locomotion control via RF control for an un-tethered cyborg.

FY 2009 Plans:
- Create a functional model of the entire mammalian object recognition pathway that is biologically valid and suitable for translation to algorithm development.
- Apply protein design methodology to: 1) perform region-specific nitration chemistry, and 2) develop a protein that inhibits the activity of influenza by preferential binding.
- Develop a fast high-throughput chemistry-based technique for determining biomolecule structures at sub-A resolution (better than X-ray cyrstallography) in solution.
- Optimize MEMS components for locomotion control, communications and power generation to consume less power and to reduce size, weight and cost.

	FY 2007	FY 2008	FY 2009
Human Assisted Neural Devices	10.500	12.000	15.000

(U) The Human Assisted Neural Devices program will develop the scientific foundation for <u>understanding the language of the brain for</u> application to a variety of emerging DoD challenges, including improving performance on the battlefield and returning active duty military to their units. This will require an understanding of neuroscience, significant computational efforts, and new material design and implementation. Key advances expected from this research include the ability to improve decision making in a variety of DoD applications including <u>imagery analysis</u>. In addition, this thrust will provide an understanding of how the brain adapts as it learns. This understanding will be translated into improved training approaches that allow transition from novices to expert in military tasks such as marksmanship to be accomplished with minimum effort and time.

Oct 2007

Working with flies allows researchers the opportunity to study specific behavioral or physiologic characteristics that would be very difficult to study in humans due to complexity in human physiology. The researchers examined families of fruit flies with unique sleep/wake characteristics in their experimental paradigm. They discovered flies that did not require as much sleep, but that still were able to perform normally on a task. These were simple behavioral tasks (for flies) like danger avoidance. These "sleep deprivation resistant flies" were used to identify the specific biochemical mechanisms of sleep deprivation resistance in flies.[1] Some of these mechanisms have been verified in rodents. The group also investigated migrating birds to try to deduce how and why birds can function with limit amounts of sleep, without performance degradation.

---

[1] Cirelli C, Bushey D, Hill S, Huber R, Kreber R, Ganetzsky B, Tononi G. Reduced sleep in Drosophila Shaker mutants. *Nature*, 434: 1087-1092, 2005a. See also http://ntp.neuroscience.wisc.edu/faculty/cirelli.html and http://ntp.neuroscience.wisc.edu/faculty/tononi.html for additional publications.

The results of these studies have been scientifically important. Investigators have discovered the detailed biochemistry of what happens to brain cells after sleep deprivation. Similar changes may also occur in forms of dementia.

Another researcher used functional Magnetic Resonance Imaging (FMRI) to image the brain of human subjects while performing a standard memory task. Researchers were able to identify differences in brain regions that were activated during the task and the individual variations in the degree of activation. After baseline imaging, the same subjects were then sleep deprived asked to perform the same memory task. The people that performed poorly on the in the task had a lower degree of activation in the brain regions used in the task after sleep deprivation. Investigators demonstrated that some subjects were able to maintain their level of performance while others could not perform as well after a lower amount of sleep. These differences in performance could be explained by differences in the use of brain "neural networks" as documented by non-invasive neuroimaging (FMRI). Transcranial magnetic stimulation may provide the ability to non-pharmacologically maintain function of these neural networks that are altered by sleep-deprivation.[2]

The research showed that people that seem to enlist more areas of their brain to perform a task before sleep deprivation seem to do better on the same task after sleep deprivation. The hypothesis is that when individuals are sleep-deprived it decreases the appropriate enlistment of task specific regions in the brain. People who are more "naturally" sleep-resistant have more available brain activation "in reserve" that they can utilize to perform a task well even in sleep-deprived conditions. People that have lower overall activation at baseline on a task fared more poorly on task performance after sleep deprivation. This work adds to the mounting evidence that function after sleep deprivation varies widely based on individual differences. The work suggests that individual differences are significant when designing any sleep deprivation countermeasure.

---

[2] Habeck C, Rakitin B, Moeller J, Scarmeas N, Zarahn E, Brown T, Stern Y. An event-related FMRI study of the neurobehavioral impact of sleep deprivation on performance of a delayed-match-to-sample task. *Cognitive Brain Research*, 18 (2004) 306-321. http://www.cumc.columbia.edu/dept/sergievsky/cnd/pdfs/AnEventRelatedFMRIStudy.pdf

DARPA also investigated how ampakines impact sleep deprivation. Ampakines are a compound that interact with AMPA receptors in the brain. Ampakines are of interest for preventing sleep deprivation because they seem to have a very specific effect on select regions of the brain that are affected by sleep deprivation, rather than the very general effect that current stimulants such as caffeine and amphetamines have on the entire nervous system. Researchers compared performance at baseline, and after sleep deprivation in a "delayed match to sample" memory task (DMS). Efficacy of ampakines was compared to currently used fatigue countermeasures such as caffeine, modafinil and ephedra in animal models. In preliminary animal studies, an ampakine known as CX717 was shown to restore one of the major biochemical changes associated with sleep deprivation, without having any typical stimulant side-effects.[3] DARPA and the Army next sponsored a study looking at the effet ampakines have on humans in a shift-work paradigm. In the study, CX717 did not reverse the effects of degraded performance and alertness from the simulated night shifts.[4]

Any therapeutic with investigations sponsored by DARPA must meet the same rigorous safety and efficacy standards, and FDA approval, as any civilian medication. These include studies which prove safety in animals after both short-term and long-term administration, and in doses orders of magnitude higher than those to be given to humans. The developer company must also prove safety in human studies to the satisfaction of the FDA and study investigators before compounds are even considered for DARPA clinical trials. All human clinical trials must also be approved by the local Institutional Review Board. Studies in Preventing Sleep Deprivation must also undergo a second level of review by any Army Human Studies Review Board. DoD Directives mandate that all studies adhere to the Common Rule.

---

[3] Facilitation of Task Performance and Removal of the Effects of Sleep Deprivation by an Ampakine (CX717) in Nonhuman Primates, by Porrino, LJ, Daunais, JB, Rogers, GA, Hampson, RE, Deadwyler, SA, Department of Physiology and Pharmacology, Wake Forest University Health Sciences, Winston-Salem, North Carolina, United States of America. PLoS Biol. 2005 August 23;3(9). http://nootropics.com/ampakines/cx717.htm

[4] Ampakine (CX717) Effects on Performance and Alertness During Simulated Night Shift Work, by Wesensten, Nancy J.; Reichardt, Rebecca M.; Balkin, Thomas J. Aviation, Space, and Environmental Medicine, Volume 78, Number 10, October 2007, pp. 937-943(7). http://www.ingentaconnect.com/content/asma/asem/2007/00000078/00000010/art00004

Exhibit R-2, RDT&E Budget Item Justification			Date: June 2001
APPROPRIATION/BUDGET ACTIVITY	R-1 ITEM NOMENCLATURE		
97 0400 4900/07	Foreign Counterintelligence Activities 0305127V		

COST (in Millions)	FY2000	FY2001	FY2002
Smallland Miscellaneous Grant	0.436	0.439	0.664

A. Mission Description and Budget Item Justification

The DoD Polygraph Institute administers the RDT&E funds contained in the DSS budget. The mission to complete Congressionally mandated research and function as the governments central research facility for deception research is accomplished via the following strategic objectives: (a) evaluate the validity of psychophysiological detection of deception (PDD) techniques used by the Department of Defense (DoD); (b) investigate countermeasures and anticountermeasures; and (c) conduct developmental research on PDD techniques, instruments, and analytic methods. In addition to these congressional mandated missions, the DoDPI Research program is investigating alternative measures, technology, and analysis techniques such as voice analysis, thermal imaging, pulse transit time, visual activity, electroencephalography, electromyography, vagal tone, electrocardiology, high definition-ERP, fMDI, and laser technologies. Proposals in this area clearly identify and support a nexus between the proposed work and the detection of deception.

In January 1999, DoDPI began an effort to enhance its presence in the scientific, academic, and technological communities. This is in response to the need for more advanced technical expertise. This initiative seeks to give the DoDPI a research workforce that is competitive with the best minds from the complex cerebral worlds of academia, and the emerging technologies. Moreover, these partnerships seek to take advantage of the highest quality University labs and industrial technology that may have solutions to our subjects of interest. While the Institute is interested in, and will support basic research, the majority of our funding will be awarded to proposals describing applied research that is of immediate use to the PDD community. The research topics of interest have been divided into the categories of Special Projects, Emerging Alternative Technology, Applied Topics, PDD Data Analyses, and Deterrence.

B. Program Change Summary

	FY2000	FY2001	FY2002
FY2001 President's Budget	0.436	0.444	0.464
Government-wide Rescissions		(0.005)	
General Increase			0.200
FY2002 President's Budget	0.436	0.439	0.664

C. Other Program Funding Summary

D. Acquisition Strategy: N/A

E. Schedule Profile: There are no scheduled acquisition, program, T&E, or contract milestones.

Dr. Eric Eisenstadt
Defense Sciences Office (DSO)
Brain Machine Interface

Our office director, Michael Goldblatt, briefly touched upon the Agency's bio vision and its four components: enhancing system performance, protecting human assets, enhancing human performance, and developing new tools for biology.

As we bring this brief overview of the Defense Sciences Office to a close, I'm pleased to have the opportunity to describe our newest and boldest initiative in human performance enhancement—the Brain Machine Interface. This program exemplifies how the office coalesce its expertise in materials, biology, and mathematics to create imaginative new opportunities that live at the interface of multiple disciplines.

Picture a time when humans see in the UV and IR portions of the electromagnetic spectrum, or hear speech on the noisy flight deck of an aircraft carrier; or when soldiers communicate by thought alone. Imagine a time when the human brain has its own wireless modem so that instead of acting on thoughts, warfighters have thoughts that act. Later during DARPATech, you will hear from IPTO about efforts to create intelligent machines.

Our Brain Machine Interface Program is about giving machine-like capabilities to intelligence, asking the brain to accommodate synthetic devices, and learning how to control those devices much the way we control our arms and legs today. Our path to realizing this vision is an interdisciplinary one—drawing from DARPA's foundation investments, combining the test of materials science, mathematics and, of course, biology.

The brain's performance is dynamic and amazing. It contains perhaps as many as 100 trillion connections; this is vastly more than the mere 55 million transistors on a Pentium 4 chip. Understanding how these connections are used to process information and control behavior is one of the great challenges of our time. DARPA is exploring the brain from a number of dimensions, from pharmacology and physiology to learning and behavior.

Several efforts are looking at improving the ability of the brain to process and retain data either by improving knowledge visualization or by active feedback and monitoring of the brain's ability to capture information and record data to memory. Other efforts are evaluating target sites and molecules for pharmacological intervention in cognitive processes.

Several programs are drawing on DARPA's strength in material science to develop devices that are orders of magnitude denser than those currently available. And, most important, several initiatives and leveraging DoD's historical ability to locate the data within noisy environments. Our unique signal processing capabilities will be deployed to help us decipher the language of the brain as we learn to record the chatter of millions of neurons communicating with one another in the language of action potentials, local field potentials, and chemical signals.

Beginning almost 2 years ago, *Science and Nature* began featuring articles from a project in Alan Rudolph's Biological Systems Program that reveal that honeybees translate optical flow data into spatial coordinates as a way to communicate the location of a food source to their hivernates. So insects use optical flow processing strategies in motion detection to navigate with high maneuverability and speed when chasing targets, avoiding collisions, and finding reproductive makers.

We have mimicked this capability in silicon by engineering microchips that control small, unmanned vehicles with the maneuverability of insects. We have demonstrated an autonomous helicopter, which can hover and do terrain following and collision avoidance of high speeds using optical flow. We also plan on using the chip in a 1-centimeter long microchemical flying insect.

And finally, to get the most bangs for our buck, we have just begun to partner with the Navy at China Lake to place a biomimetic seeker on a hydrorocket. We are betting that a fairly low-resolution rocket using biologically inspired signal processing algorithms on the front end could be used to find and hit a moving target with greater accuracy.

The harbinger of our Brain Machine Interface Program began with our foray into the creation of a wireless brain modem for a freely moving rat. Here, we are able to create, in real-time, at a standoff distance, interactions with the brain to allow us to control the motor behavior of a rat. The objective of this effort is to use remote teleoperation via direct interconnections with the brain. These implants can last in the brain for a year or more and are used to steer the rat by providing positive rewards to the rats (or other animal systems) as they perform in accordance with certain desires. As this movie of Roborat demonstrates, he can be directed to move in unusual and quite capable ways.

Here, Roborat is demonstrating that we can obtain the kind of mobility and dynamic capability in locomotion that could be very useful in search and rescue of other surveillance opportunities. Most roboticists can appreciate that there is nothing in their labs that can move like this.

The next obvious move in this direction is to use higher density interconnects to create and collect information from the brain in other regions associated with sensory input. Why? As just one example, imagine if we could plug into the olfactory cortex region of the brain and interpret from a distance what an animal smells. Is that cocaine? Explosives? A rat-fearing human?

You may have read recently about clinical experiments using a retinal implant that utilized a prosthetic device carrying an array of only 16 elements that enabled blind patients to discriminate light from dark and shadows. But to prove a blind person with the ability to see images, prosthetic vision devices require much higher resolution. We are about to find out what happens when you plug high-density interconnects into the visual sensory system.

Another project in the Controlled Biological System Program—a collaborative effort between investigators at John Hopkins University and the Naval Research Laboratory—developed a nanochannel glass array containing 3,200 elements that can communicate with the retina compared to the 16 that were used in the current experimental devices. Images from a digital camera will be transferred via the high-density nanochannel array to the retina and to the brain, where an image will be created. Wires are now used to transport images from the digital camera to the nanoarray. In the future, however, images will be transmitted wirelessly. We anticipate that within a year or so, the new high-resolution device will be in human clinical trials.

These and other projects involving high density interconnects with the brain seduced DARPA to further investigate interactions with other regions of the brain. We are creating new high-density interconnects for brain machine interfaces that will allow us to monitor the brain patterns associated with a wide variety of behaviors and activities relevant to DoD.

And now we are equipped to aggressively begin moving beyond acting on thoughts to having thoughts that act. Hence, the recently initiated Brain Machine Interface Program. This program was launched to demonstrate the use of brain activity to command, control, actuate, and communicate with the world directly through brain interfaces. Initially these interactions are with peripheral devices, but ultimately it may be interaction with another brain. The first peripheral devices were robotic arms.

Three research groups supported by DARPA recently demonstrated that when a monkey is trained to do a peripheral motor task, such as reaching for a piece of fruit, the executive command activity associated with that behavior can be intercepted and then used to control artificial devices that execute the same movements. In a closed loop, the monkey can learn to drive a peripheral device—or a curse on a screen—using only its brain's executive motor commands.

We are pushing hard to study how to provide the sensory feedback directly to the brain of the experience of that peripheral device. The Brain Machine Interface Program is asking the brain to accommodate synthetic devices and learn how to control these devices much the way we control our arms and legs.

There a number of imprisonment new materials and signal-processing questions that we will be asking in terms of controlling more complex kinds of DoD-related technologies, such as exoskeletons or airframes. Additionally, even the most aggressive proponents of the brain machine interface vision recognize the long-term need to be able to noninvasively capture the brain's internal communications, to listen and understand without having to implant hardware.

Who knows . . . if we can eavesdrop on the brain, maybe we can sort out deceit from honesty, truth from fiction. What a lie detector that would be!

The skills required to make this happen—math, biology, material science, physics, and imagination—represent many of the strengths of the Defense Sciences Office.

Thank you.

U.S. Department of Justice

United States Attorney
Eastern District of New York

TAM:RWS:jac

271 Cadman Plaza East
Brooklyn, New York 11201

February 1, 2010

VIA ELECTRONIC FILING AND HAND DELIVERY

Honorable Joseph F. Bianco
United States District Court Judge
Eastern District of New York
924 Federal Plaza
Central Islip, New York 11722

> Re: *Gilbert Roman v. DARPA*
> Civil Action No. CV-09-5633 (E.D.N.Y.) (Bianco, J.) (Wall, J.)

Dear Judge Bianco:

This office represents the defendant in the above-referenced matter. I write to respectfully request a sixty (60) day extension of time, from February 8, 2010, to April 9, 2010, to answer, move, or otherwise respond to plaintiff's complaint, which seeks an order compelling the release of records pursuant to the Freedom of Information Act. This is the defendant's first request for an extension, which is necessary because I understand that defendant will be sending plaintiff documents responsive to his requests shortly. The requested extension will give plaintiff time to review this information and determine whether this matter needs to proceed. I have conferred with the *pro se* plaintiff on this matter and he has consented to this request.

Thank you for your consideration of this request.

Very truly yours,

BENTON J. CAMPBELL
United States Attorney

By: s/ *Robert W. Schumacher* (electronically filed)
ROBERT W. SCHUMACHER
Assistant U.S. Attorney
(718) 254-6035

cc: Gilbert Roman, *Pro Se* Plaintiff (Via First Class Mail)
95-25 77th Street
Ozone Park, NY 11416

DECLARATION OF SERVICE

Jennifer Casado, hereby declares and states as follows:

That on the 1st day of February, 2010 I caused to be mailed by First Class Mail, from 610 Federal Plaza, 5th Floor, Central Islip, New York, the following:

LETTER REQUESTING SIXTY DAY EXTENSION OF TIME
TO ANSWER OR OTHERWISE MOVE

Of which the annexed is a true copy contained in a securely enclosed postpaid wrapper directed to the person(s) at the place(s) and address(es) as follows:

Gilbert Roman
Plaintiff, pro se
95-25 77th Street
Ozone Park, NY 11416

The undersigned affirms under penalty of perjury that the foregoing is true and correct.

Dated: Central Islip, New York
          February 1, 2010

S/ Jennifer Casado
JENNIFER CASADO

Motions

2:09-cv-05633-JFB -WDW Roman v. DARPA
NPROSE

U.S. District Court

Eastern District of New York

Notice of Electronic Filing

The following transaction was entered by Schumacher, Robert on 2/1/2010 at 2:30 PM EST and filed on 2/1/2010

Case Name: Roman v. DARPA
Case Number: 2:09-cv-05633-JFB -WDW
Filer: DARPA
Document Number: 7

Docket Text:
Letter MOTION for Extension of Time to File Answer *or otherwise move from February 8, 2010 to April 9, 2010* by DARPA. (Attachments: # (1) Affidavit of Service) (Schumacher, Robert)

2:09-cv-05633-JFB -WDW Notice has been electronically mailed to:

Robert W. Schumacher , II   robert.schumacher@usdoj.gov, Jennifer.casado@usdoj.gov

2:09-cv-05633-JFB -WDW Notice will not be electronically mailed to:

Gilbert Roman
95-25 77th St.
Ozone Park, NY 11416

The following document(s) are associated with this transaction:

Document description: Main Document
Original filename: n/a
Electronic document Stamp:
[STAMP NYEDStamp_ID=875559751 [Date=2/1/2010] [FileNumber=4975947-0] [
0f06c0749f2b6275d2210c315df1b10e8219529327c42e058adcfb81acbbd9089c5e06
79c51161ba9743afd3753b6450ebe42567e810b89d9b83c08df52e20be]]
Document description: Affidavit of Service
Original filename: n/a
Electronic document Stamp:
[STAMP NYEDStamp_ID=875559751 [Date=2/1/2010] [FileNumber=4975947-1] [
9460cd368e896c37053302f8ef3f0de4c95a9b7a754d3f67fbca2530b9adbb4365a15a
ee2b81fcc1870d5095217709ae8a0fe7f9a0968c18faa2251197ae02e6]]

NATIONAL SECURITY AGENCY EXHIBIT

These are the FOIA requests I made to the NSA. In one, they refused to answer, and the other, they claimed an executive order not to answer. I asked for satellite surveillance records for New York and New Jersey and satellite time logs. This information will prove if any illegal activities are taking place by monitoring Americans in America. I was denied access by the courts so far.

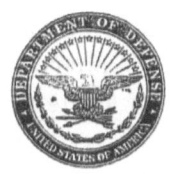

NATIONAL SECURITY AGENCY
CENTRAL SECURITY SERVICE

FORT GEORGE G. MEADE, MARYLAND 20755-6000

FOIA Case: 53444
28 August 2007

Mr. Gilbert Roman
P.O. Box 37023
Elmont, NY 11003

Dear Mr. Roman:

This responds to your Freedom of Information Act (FOIA) request of 27 July 2007, which was received by this office on 3 August 2007, for the following:

1. The satellite time logs for satellites focused on New York and New Jersey State from January 1985 to January 1991.
2. The total amount of hours a satellite was focused on New York and New Jersey State.

Your letter has been assigned Case Number 53444. Please refer to this case number when contacting us about your request.

From purposes of this request and based on the information you provided in your letter, you are considered an "all other" requester. As such, you are allowed 2 hours of search and the duplication of 100 pages at no cost. There are no assessable fees for this request. Your request has been processes under the provisions of the FOIA.

We have determined that the fact of the existence or non-existence of the materials you request in a currently and properly classified matter in accordance with Executive Order 12958, as amended. Thus, your request is denied pursuant to the first exemption of the FOIA which provides that the FOIA does not apply to matters that are specifically authorized under criteria established by an Executive order to be kept secret in the interest of national defense or foreign relations and are, in fact properly classified pursuant to such Executive Order.

In addition, this Agency is authorized by various statutes to protect certain information concerning its activities. The third exemption of the FOIA provides for the withholding of information specifically protected from disclosure by statue. Thus, your request is also denied because the fact of the existence and non-existence of the information is exempted from disclosure pursuant to the third exemption. The specific statutes applicable in this case are Title 18 U.S. Code 798; Title 50 U.S. Code 403-1(i); and Section 6, Public Law 86-36 (50 U.S. Code 402 note).

As your request is being denied, you are hereby advised of this Agency's appeal procedures. Any person denied access to information may file an appeal to the NSA/CSS Freedom of information Act Appeal Authority. The appeal must be postmarked no later than 60 calendar days of the date of the initial denial letter. The appeal shall be in writing addressed to the NSA/CSSS FOIA Appeal Authority (DJ4), National Security Agency, 9800 Savage Road STE 6248, Fort George G. Meade, MD 20755-6248. The appeal shall reference the adverse determination and shall contain, in sufficient detail and particularity, the grounds upon which the requester believes that the determination is unwarranted. The NSA/CSS FOIA Appeal Authority will endeavor to respond to the appeal within 20 working days after receipt, absent any unusual circumstances.

Sincerely,

RHEA D. SIERS
Deputy Associate Director for Policy

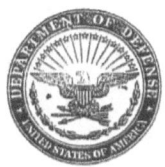

NATIONAL SECURITY SERVICE

FORT GEORGE G. MEADE, MARYLAND 20755-6000

Case No. 53444/Appeal No. 3280
3 October 2007

Mr. Gilbert Roman
P.O. Box 37023
Elmont, NY 11003

Dear Mr. Roman:

This replies to your letter, dated 12 September 2007, appealing the National Security Agency's (NSA) denial of your request under the Freedom of Information Act (FOIA). You had requested the satellite time logs for satellites focused on New York and New Jersey State from January 1985 to January 1991; and the total amount of hours a satellite was focused on New York and New Jersey State. Your original request, the Deputy Associate Director of Policy's response to you, and your letter of appeal have been reviewed. As a result of this review, I have concluded that the appropriate response to your request is to continue to neither confirm nor deny the existence of the materials you request.

The existence or non-existence of the information you requested is exempt from disclosure pursuant to 5 U.S. § 552(b)(1), which protects properly classified information. I have determined that any substantive response to your request would tend to confirm or deny specific activities. The fact of the existence or non-existence of such information is a properly classified matter under Executive Order 12958, as amended, since it meets the specific criteria for classification established in Sections 1.4(c) and (g) of the Order. When such classification is warranted, Section 3.6(a) allows an agency to respond by declining to confirm or deny the existence or non-existence of responsive records.

Further, the fact of the existence or non-existence of the records requested is also exempt pursuant to 5 U.S.C. § 552(b)(3), which permits withholding of matters specifically exempted from disclosure by statute. The applicable statutory provisions with regard to the existence or non-existence

25

of the records requested are: Section 6 of the National Security Act of 1959 (Public Law 86-36, 50 U.S.C. § 402 note), which provides that no law shall be construed to require the disclosure of the organization, personnel, functions, or activities of the National Security Agency; 50 U.S.C. § 403-1(i)(1), which requires the protection of intelligence sources and methods from unauthorized disclosure; and 18 U.S.C. § 798, which prohibits the release of information concerning classified communications intelligence activities except to those persons authorized to receive such information.

Since this response may be construed as a denial of your appeal, you are hereby advised of your right pursuant to 5 U.S.C. § 552(a)(4)(B) to seek judicial review of my decision in the United States District Court, in the district in which you reside, in which you have your principal place of business, in which the Agency records are situated (U.S. District Court of Maryland), or in the District of Columbia.

Sincerely,

JOHN C. INGLIS
Freedom of Information Act/Privacy Act
Appeals Authority

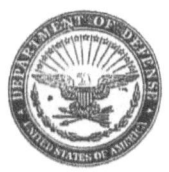

NATIONAL SECURITY AGENCY
CENTRAL SECURITY SERVICE

FORT GEORGE G. MEADE, MARYLAND 20755-6000

FOIA Case: 54314
20 December 2007

Mr. Gilbert Roman
1476 L Street
Elmont, NY 11003

Dear Mr. Roman:

This is in response to your Freedom of Information Act (FOIA) request of 4 December 2007, which was received by this office on 11 December 2007, for satellite surveillance records covering New York and New Jersey for the period of January 1987 until December 2007. Your request has been assigned Case Number 54314. There is certain information relating to this processing about which the FOIA and applicable Department of Defense (DoD) and NSA/CSS regulations require we inform you.

For purposes of this request and based on the information you provided in your letter, you are considered an "all over" requester. You must pay for search time in excess of 2 hours and duplication in excess of 100 pages. There are no assessable fees for this request.

This Agency has already complied with the FOIA and on 28 August 2007 provided a response to you concerning this subject matter (FOIA Case 53444), which was upheld on appeal (Appeal Case Number 3280). As stated in our previous response letters to you, the fact of the existence or non-existence of satellite surveillance records covering New York and New Jersey is both classified and protected from disclosure by statute. This would be true for any time period. This request is considered a duplicate submission of your previous request and appeal and, therefore, will be administratively closed. Be advised that further requests from you on this subject matter, regardless of time period stated in your requests, will not be processed under the Freedom of Information act Act.

Sincerely,

Marianne Stupar
for
PAMELA N. PHILLIPS
Chief
FOIA/PA Office

A CALL TO NOTICE

I call upon all U.S. citizens to question how this technology is being used. We must take action and write or elected officials. Remember early Venitian history—no one person or group was allowed to have absolute power. This technology gives monitoring an absolute ungoverned power.

On the next page, we will find one of the ways FMRI technology has been used in the courts system. Will this technology be used for justice to clear court calendars one day? God only knows. I do know that if not made public, we will be left in the dark on how it is really being used.

FMRI scans used in murder-trial sentencing

November 25, 2009 by Lin Edwards

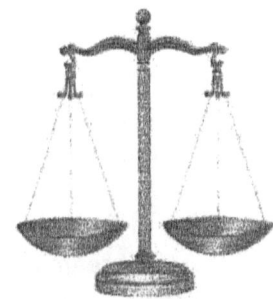

Scale of justice. Image: *Wikipedia*

(PhysOrg.com)—Functional Magnetic Resonance Imaging (FMRI) scans have been used, possibly for the first time, in the sentencing phase of a murder trial in Chicago in the US.

The defendant, Brian Dugan, was convicted for the 1983 kidnapping, rape and murder of a 10-year-old girl, Jeanine Nicarico. Dugan had pleaded guilty in July this year, while serving life sentences for two other murders. Prosecutors at the trial asked for the death penalty to be imposed.

The defense lawyers believed Dugan had suffered from a mental illness—psychopathy—from birth and asked for FMRI scans to be presented as evidence in the sentencing phase. Lead defense attorney Steve Greeberg said the FMRI scans indicated Dugan had a brain disorder in keeping with psychopathy, and his mental illness meant his ability to control his psychopathic urges was reduced.

Dugan had been given a standard diagnostic test for psychopathy and scored 37 out of a possible 40, which placed him in the 99.5th percentile, according to neuroscientist Kent Kiehl of the University of Mexico, who was an expert witness for the defense.

Kiehl runs FMRI and other brain scans on inmates in prisons in New Mexico, as they perform a series of activities, including tests involving moral reasoning. Kiehl testified that Dugan's FMRI scans showed similar features to those of other psychopaths.

An expert witness for the prosecution, Jonathan Brodie of New York University, said the evidence presented by the scans was irrelevant since they could not indicate Dugan's thought processes in 1983, when the murder was committed.

After 10 hours of deliberation the jury returned with the death sentence, apparently after a change of mind in at least one juror who had wanted Dugan to receive a life sentence instead. Greenberg said the last minute change was highly irregular, as he is planning to appeal.

In previous cases PET scans have been used as evidence of brain disorders, but the Dugan case is believed to be the first in which FMRI scans have been used. Professor Hank Greely of Standford Law School said the standards required for evidence in the sentencing phase were less stringent than during the trial, especially in capital cases when the law makes special dispensation to allow the defendant to introduce almost any evidence that might save him from the death penalty. (PhysOrg.com)

NATIONAL RECONNAISSANCE OFFICE EXHIBIT

I have made many FOIA request to the NRO over the years. I now can claim that lies have been made. Justice has been obstructed, and maybe other claims later on. Read through the forms and see for yourself. I also requested FOIA processing forms for my request. No search time is entered, and how could they have searched without search time? And only low-level searches were made. FMRI technology must be in top secret—level files, and top secret—level files must be searched. Why do the courts continue to ignore all these facts?

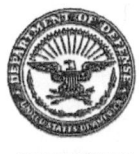

OFFICE OF THE ASSISTANT SECRETARY OF DEFENSE
1400 DEFENSE PENTAGON
WASHINGTON, DC 20301 1400

PUBLIC AFFAIRS

06 SEP 1996

Ref: 96-F-1693
96-P-0117

Mr. Gilbert Roman

Dear Mr. Roman:

This responds to your August 16, 1996, Freedom of
Information Act (FOIA) and Privacy Act request received in this
Directorate on August 22, 1996.

Due to the size and complexity of the Department of Defense
(DoD), there is no central repository for all DoD records. This
Directorate is responsible for responding to requests for records
of the components of the Office of the Secretary of Defense and
the Joint Staff (OSD/JS). The several components of the DoD,
including the military departments and separate defense agencies,
operate their own Freedom of Information offices to respond to
requests for records for which they are responsible. These
procedures are provided in DoD regulation 5400.7-R, as published
at 32 CFR 286.

The information you have requested, if it exists, would be
under the cognizance of the National Reconnaissance Office (NRO)
Your request has been forwarded to them at the following address
for their action and direct reply to you:

National Reconnaissance Office/FOIA Officer
1040 Defense Pentagon
Room 4C1000
Washington, DC 20301-1040

Please direct any questions regarding this action to
Lieutenant Commander Lewis Guerin, USN, at (703) 697-2716.

Sincerely,

A. H. Passarella
Director
Freedom of Information
and Security Review

31

FREEDOM OF INFORMATION PROCESSING

CASE NUMBER: _F96-0054_ DATE COMPLETED: _____ OFFICE: _OS/PSD_

(SEARCH)(REVIEW)   *No search time entered*   (SEARCH)(REVIEW)

(IS2-4; GS-03-08; E1-E9):

    TOTAL HOURS _____ _____ X $12.00 (PER HOUR) = _____ _____

(GS/M-09-15; 01-06):

    TOTAL HOURS _____ _____ X $25.00 (PER HOUR) = _____ _____

(GS/M-16 AND ABOVE; 07-010):

    TOTAL HOURS _____ _____ X $45.00 (PER HOUR) = _____ _____

COMPUTER SEARCH:

    MACHINE HRS _____ _____ X $10.00 (ON-LINE) = _____ _____

    MACHINE HRS _____ _____ X $25.00 (BATCH) = _____ _____

PRINTED RECORDS (FORMS, PUBLICATIONS, REPORTS):

    TOTAL PAGES _____ X .02 = _____

REPRODUCTION: (ER/FOIA USE ONLY)

    # OF PAGES REPRODUCED _____ X .15 (PER PAGE) = _____

FOR - INFORMATION ACCESS & RELEASE CENTER - INTERNAL USE ONLY

SEARCH FEES _____ OUTSTANDING FEES _____

REVIEW FEES _____

REPRODUCTION FEES _____ TOTAL CHARGED TO DATE _____

TOTAL CHARGED _____ FEE CATEGORY

TOTAL PAID _____ ☐ COMMERCIAL
    ☐ EDUCATION/MEDIA
    ☐ OTHER

DATE PAID _____ FEES WAIVED: _____ YES _____ NO

NRO FOIA Processing Form

FREEDOM OF INFORMATION PROCESSING

CASE NUMBER: _F96-0054_ DATE COMPLETED: _____ OFFICE: __OS__

(SEARCH) (REVIEW) *Search time entered* (SEARCH) (REVIEW)

(IS2-4; GS-03-08; E1-E9):

    TOTAL HOURS ___1___ _____ X $12.00 (PER HOUR) = ___12.00___

(GS/M-09-15; 01-06):

    TOTAL HOURS _____ _____ X $25.00 (PER HOUR) = _____ _____

(GS/M-16 AND ABOVE; 07-010):

    TOTAL HOURS _____ _____ X $45.00 (PER HOUR) = _____ _____

COMPUTER SEARCH:

    MACHINE HRS _____ _____ X $10.00 (ON-LINE) = _____ _____

    MACHINE HRS _____ _____ X $25.00 (BATCH) = _____ _____

PRINTED RECORDS (FORMS, PUBLICATIONS, REPORTS):

    TOTAL PAGES _____ X .02 = _____

REPRODUCTION: (ER/FOIA USE ONLY)

    # OF PAGES REPRODUCED _____ X .15 (PER PAGE) = _____

FOR - INFORMATION ACCESS & RELEASE CENTER - INTERNAL USE ONLY

SEARCH FEES _____ OUTSTANDING FEES _____

REVIEW FEES _____

REPRODUCTION FEES _____ TOTAL CHARGED TO DATE _____

TOTAL CHARGED _____

FEE CATEGORY
☐ COMMERCIAL
☐ EDUCATION/MEDIA
☐ OTHER

TOTAL PAID _____

DATE PAID _____ FEES WAIVED: _____ YES _____ NO

Notice only the lowest level was searched

33

FREEDOM OF INFORMATION ACT (FOIA) REQUEST
FOIA NUMBER
10-F-96-277

Date Rec'd	To Prog. Office	To FOIA	To Code G	To FOIA	To Requester	Suspense
8/28/96						9/7/96

FROM: **Gilbert Roman**

ACTION OFFICE: **COB**

THE ATTACHED REQUEST IS TO BE RESPONDED TO ONLY BY THE FOIA OFFICE. PLEASE RETURN INFO REQUESTED TO ROOM 8M78. IF YOU REQUIRE ANY ASSISTANCE, PLEASE CONTACT PAT REIP-DICE (358-1764) OR DONNA CLAVELLI (358-1762).

COMMENTS:

No Information available

No Search time
NASA FOIA FORM

ACTION OFFICE   LEGAL TECHNICIAN   ATTORNEY

SEARCH
TIME (Qtr Hrs)   GRADE   TIME (Qtr Hrs)   GRADE   TIME (Qtr Hrs)   GRADE

_____   _____   _____

_____   _____   _____

NAME   NAME   NAME

NOTE: ALL FOIA REQUESTS MUST BE ROUTED BETWEEN OFFICES ON A HAND-CARRY BASIS. THE NORMAL MAIL SYSTEM WILL NOT BE USED. THE LAW REQUIRES THAT THE REQUEST BE ANSWERED WITHIN 10 WORKING DAYS OF RECEIPT. COGNIZANT OFFICES ARE EXPECTED TO RESPOND BY THE SUSPENSE DATE.

THIS IS TO CERTIFY THAT ALL PROGRAM FILES PERTAINING TO THE FOIA REQUEST HAVE BEEN SEARCHED AND COPIES OF ALL DOCUMENTS LOCATED HAVE BEEN FURNISHED TO THE FOIA OFFICE.

_____   12   COB
SIGNATURE OF INDIVIDUAL CERTIFYING ABOVE   GRADE   CODE

FREEDOM OF INFORMATION ACT (FOIA) REQUEST
FOIA NUMBER
10-F- 98-7

Rec'd	To Prog. Office	To FOIA	To Code G	To FOIA	To Requester	Suspense
10/6/97	10/6/97					10/20/97

Gilbert Roman

ACTION OFFICE: 4 (S), U

ATTACHED REQUEST IS TO BE RESPONDED TO ONLY BY THE FOIA OFFICE. PLEASE RETURN TO REQUESTED TO ROOM 8M78. IF YOU REQUIRE ANY ASSISTANCE, PLEASE CONTACT RIP-DICE (358-1764) OR DONNA CLAVELLI (358-1762).

COMMENTS:

Code S has no input
5 mins of search time
1 level of security clearance searched

ACTION OFFICE		LEGAL TECHNICIAN		ATTORNEY	
TIME (Qtr Hrs)	GRADE	TIME (Qtr Hrs)	GRADE	TIME (Qtr Hrs)	GRADE
5 mins	9				

Cheryl L. Ellis 10/7

| | NAME | NAME |

NOTE ALL FOIA REQUESTS MUST BE ROUTED BETWEEN OFFICES ON A HAND-CARRY BASIS. THE NORMAL MAIL SYSTEM WILL NOT BE USED. THE LAW REQUIRES THAT THE REQUEST BE ANSWERED WITHIN 10 WORKING DAYS OF RECEIPT. COGNIZANT OFFICES ARE EXPECTED TO RESPOND BY THE SUSPENSE DATE.

THIS IS TO CERTIFY THAT ALL PROGRAM FILES PERTAINING TO THE FOIA REQUEST HAVE BEEN SEARCHED AND COPIES OF ALL DOCUMENTS LOCATED HAVE BEEN FURNISHED TO THE FOIA OFFICE.

Cheryl L. Ellis

SIGNATURE OF INDIVIDUAL CERTIFYING ABOVE	9	S
	GRADE	CODE

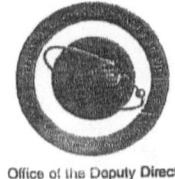

NATIONAL RECONNAISSANCE OFFICE
14675 Lee Road
Chantilly, VA 20151-1715

Office of the Deputy Director

28 February 1997

Mr. Gilbert Roman

Case Number F96-0054

Dear Mr. Roman:

This is in response to your letter dated 8 January 1997. Your letter presents an appeal of the determination you received from the National Reconnaissance Office (NRO) dated 26 September Department of Defense, and referred to the NRO for direct response to you. Specifically, you requested the following records:

1. ". . . the complete biographical backgrounds on all personnel assigned to the 8X spy satellite program & US Policy on Remote Sensing Space Capabilities. The medical, scientific, & scholastic backgrounds of these gentlemen."

2. ". . . copies of any and all flyers and tapes which read (The Gov't Can read Our Minds) . . . fingerprint verification (who's fingerprints appear on these papers)."

3. ". . . any and all papers and tapes pertaining to me . . . born ??? ss#

4. ". . . the annual budget for these two programs" (8X spy satellite program & US Policy on Remote Sensing Space Capabilities).

5. ". . . how many satellites are in orbit with the technology which reads the pulses and patterns of the human brain, and converts these readings into words and sentences. This technology is built into the 8X spy satellite program and might fall under the name US Policy on Remote Sensing Space Capabilities . . . the person assigned to retrieve

this data . . . said person sign an affidavit stating his clearance . . . a list of all levels of clearance assigned to personnel."

Your appeal was presented to me as the NRO Appellate Authority. After a review of the initial determination, I have determined that we must neither confirm nor deny the existence or nonexistence of any records responsive to Items No. 1, No. 4, and No. 5 of your request. Such information, that is, whether or not any responsive records exist, would be classified for reasons of national security under Section 1.5(c) of Executive Order 12958. This denial is taken in accordance with the provisions of Title 5 U.S.C. Section 552(b) (1). By this statement, we are neither confirming nor denying that any such records exist. With respect to Items No. 2 and No. 3, the NRO has no records responsive to your request.

You are advised that you have the right to judicial review of this decision in a United States District Court in accordance with Title 5, U.S.C. Section 552.

Sincerely,

Keith R. Hall

Keith R. Hall

On February 28, 1997, NRO claimed they did not confirm nor deny the existence of technology that reads our thoughts; and on July 1, 2009, they responded with a no-records responsive to my request.

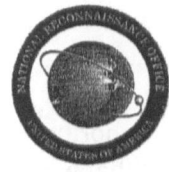

NATIONAL RECONNAISSANCE OFFICE
14675 Lee Road
Chantilly, VA 20151-1715

16 June 2009

Gilbert Roman
95-25 77th Street
Ozone Park, NY 11416

Dear Mr. Roman:

This is in response to your letter, dated 14 May 2009, received in the Information Management Services Center of the National Reconnaissance Office (NRO) on 20 May 2009, and your subsequent correspondence, dated 27 May 2009. In your 14 May letter, pursuant to the Freedom of Information Act (FOIA), you requested:

"1. . . . information on functional magnetic resonance imaging.
2. The date it was put into service.
3. The first successful report on the first person it was used on successfully."

We have accepted your request. It will be processed in accordance with the FOIA, 5 U.S.C. § 552, as amended, and the NRO Operational File Exemption, 50 U.S.C. § 432a. Unles you object, we will limit our search to NRO-originated records existing through the date of this acceptance letter.

Since we may not respond within the 20 working days stipulated by the Act, you have the right to consider this as a denial and may appeal to the NRO Appeal Review Panel. It would seem more reasonable, however, to have us continue processing your request and respond as soon as we can. You may appeal any denial of records at that time. Unless we hear from you otherwise, we will assume that you agree, and will proceed on this basis. Fees are incurred whether we find responsive records or not.

The FOIA authorizes federal agencies to assess fees for record services. Based upon the information provided, you have been placed in the "other" category of requesters, which means you are responsible for the cost of search time exceeding two hours ($44.00/hour) and reproduction fees (.15 per page) exceeding 100 pages. We will notify you if it appears that assessable fees will exceed our $25.00 minimum billing threshold.

As mentioned previously in our response letter to you, the law requires that requesters express a willingness to pay fees for this service. We have not yet received that willingness to pay from you. As a courtesy to you, in this case, we will proceed with the search up until the point that fees are incurred. You will receive the benefit of two hours of search time and 100 pages of copying. At that point, we will notify you that we have begun to incur costs and ask that you provide us with that willingness to pay fees before we continue. You may specify a limit at that time.

With regard to the issue of your 3 March 2009 request, we have been able to track the receipt of your correspondence within the NRO's Mail Processing Center on 9 March 2009. It appears, however, that the correspondence was lost or misdirected internally, and did not arrive at the proper destination for acknowledgement and processing. We apologize for the delay and inconvenience caused by this error.

If you have any questions, please call the Requester Service Center at (703) 227-9326 and reference case number F09-0063.

Sincerely,

Linda S. Hathaway
Chief, Information Access
and Release Team

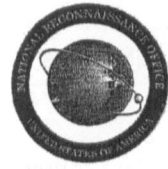

NATIONAL RECONNAISSANCE OFFICE

14675 Lee Road
Chantilly, VA 20151-1715

1 July 2009

Gilbert Roman
95-25 77th Street
Ozone Park, NY 11416

Dear Mr. Roman:

This is in response to your letter, dated 14 May 2009, received in the Information Management Services Center of the National Reconnaissance Office (NRO) on 20 May 2009, and your subsequent correspondence, dated 27 May 2009. In your 14 May letter, pursuant to the Freedom of Information Act (FOIA), you requested:

"1. . . . information on functional magnetic resonance imaging.
 2. The date it was put into service.
 3. The first successful report on the first person it was used on successfully."

Your request was processed under the FOIA, Title 5 U.S.C. § 552, as amended. A thorough search for NRO-originated records in our files and databases revealed that <u>we have no responsive records pertaining to your request</u>.

The FOIA authorizes federal agencies to assess fees for record services. Based upon the information provided, you have been placed in the "other" category of requesters, which means you are responsible for the cost of search time exceeding two hours ($44.00/hour) and reproduction fees (.15 per page) exceeding 100 pages. In this case, fees incurred in processing your request total $132.00, for 3 hours of search time in excess of the two hours provided at no cost, billed at a rate of $44.00 per hour. All fees are being waived because responsive records, if they did exist, would likely be the subject of significant public interest.

You have the right to appeal this determination by addressing your appeal to the NRO Appeal Authority, 14675 Lee Road, Chantilly, VA 20151-1715, within 60 days of the date of this letter. Should you decide to do so, please explain the basis of your appeal.

If you have any questions, please call the Requester Service Center at (703) 227-9326 and reference case number F09-0063.

Sincerely,

Linda S. Hathaway
Chief, Information Access
and Release Team

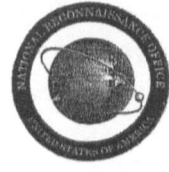

NATIONAL RECONNAISSANCE OFFICE

14675 Lee Road
Chantilly, VA 20151-1715

15 October 2009

Gilbert Roman
95-25 77th Street
Ozone Park, NY 11416

Dear Mr. Roman:

This is in response to your letter dated 12 July 2009, received in the Information Access and Release Center of the National Reconnaissance Office (NRO) on 21 July 2009, appealing our 1 July 2009 determination that the NRO has no records responsive to your 14 May 2009 request pursuant to the Freedom of Information Act for:

"1. ... information on functional magnetic resonance imaging.
2. The date it was put into service.
3. The first successful report on the first person it was used on successfully."

As the Appellate Authority, and after a complete review, I have determined that there are no National Reconnaissance Office (NRO) records responsive to your request. We have conducted reasonable searches of those components within the NRO that might have records within the parameters of your request. This action is taken in accordance with the provisions of 5 U.S.C. § 552.

You are advised that you are entitled to a judicial review of this determination in a United States District Court in accordance with 5 U.S.C. § 552.

Sincerely,

Charles Barlow

42

NATIONAL RECONNAISSANCE OFFICE
14675 Lee Road
Chantilly, VA 20151-1715

2 November 2009

Gilbert Roman
95-25 77th Street
Ozone Park, NY 11416

Remember the book *Spies, Lies and Whistleblowers*. It says that if a proper twofold entre is not done, a no-record response will be given (pages 115-116).

Dear Mr. Roman:

This is in response to your letter dated 25 October 2009, received in the Information Management Services Center of the National Reconnaissance Office (NRO) on 30 October 2009. Pursuant to the Freedom of Information Act (FOIA), you are requesting:

1) ". . . copies of all the Freedom of Information Act and/or Privacy Act of 1974 task sheets used to process my request to your agency; which you responded on July 1, 2009 and Oct. 15, 2009 . . ."
2) "Copies of the DUTY OFFICERS forms authorizing these searches to be made on July 1, 2009 and Oct. 15, 2009; Your response letters to my request for FMRI technology."
3) "Copies of the forms from the CLASSIFIED DOCUMENT RECEIPTS authorizing searches for my request for FRMI technology; which you responded on July 1, 2009 and Oct. 15, 2009."
4) "Copies of the forms from the OFFICE OF THE CLASSIFIED DOCUMENT REGISTER OF CONTROL Authorizing searches my request for FMRI technology; which you responded July 1, 2009 and Oct. 15, 2009."
5) "Copies of any and all memorandums, e-emails concerning Gilbert Roman (ME)."

We have accepted your request. It is being processed in accordance with the FOIA, 5 U.S.C. § 552, as amended, and the NRO Operational File Exemption, 50 U.S.C. § 432a. Unless you object, we will limit our search to NRO-originated records existing through the date of this acceptance letter.

Since we may not respond within the 20 working days stipulated by the Act, you have the right to consider this as a denial and may appeal to the NRO

Appeal Review Panel. It would seem more reasonable, however, to have us continue processing your request and respond as soon as we can. You may appeal any denial of records at that time. Unless we hear from you otherwise, we will assume that you agree, and will proceed on this basis.

The FOIA authorizes federal agencies to assess fees for record services. Based upon the information provided, you have been placed in the "other" category of requesters, which means you are responsible for the cost of search time exceeding two hours ($44.00/hour) and reproduction fees (.15 per page) exceeding 100 pages. Additional information about fees can be found on our website at www.nro.gov.

If your request you expressed a willingness to pay "after clearance by me." We will notify you if it appears that assessable fees will meet or exceed our $25.00 minimum billing threshold.

Regarding your request for a fee waiver, please be advised that fee waivers or reductions are granted when there is a public interest in disclosure of information, which will contribute significantly to the public's understanding of the operations or activities of the NRO. A decision to waive or reduce fees cannot be made until after any responsive documents to be disclosed have been reviewed for "public interest".

You have the right to appeal this determination by addressing your appeal to the NRO Appeal Authority, 14675 Lee Road, Chantilly, VA 20151-1715 within 60 days of the date of this letter. Should you decide to do so, please explain the basis of your appeal.

If you have any questions, please call the Requester Service Center at (703) 227-9326 and reference case number F10-0034.

Sincerely,

Stephen R. Glenn
Chief, Information Access
and Release Team

NATIONAL RECONNAISSANCE OFFICE
14675 Lee Road
Chantilly, VA 20151-1715

22 July 2009

Gilbert Roman
95-25 77th Street
Ozone Park, NY 11416

Dear Mr. Roman:

This is in response to your letter dated 12 July 2009, received in the Information Access and Release Center of the National Reconnaissance Office (NRO) on 21 July 2009. Pursuant to the Freedom of Information Act (FOIA), you are appealing the NRO's response to your request for ". . . information on functional magnetic resonance imaging . . ."

Your appeal has been accepted. We will advise you when a determination by the NRO Appeal Board has been made.

If you have any questions, please call the Requester Service Center at (703) 227-9326, and reference case number F09-0063.

Sincerely,

Linda S. Hathaway
Chief, Information Access
and Release Team

RDT&E BUDGET ITEM JUSTIFICATION SHEET (R-2 Exhibit)	DATE February 2008
APPROPRIATION/BUDGET ACTIVITY RDT&E, Defense-wide BA1 Basic Research	R-1 ITEM NOMENCLATURE Defense Research Sciences PE 0601101E, Project BLS-01

(U) Program Plans:

FY 2007 Accomplishments:
- Demonstrated neurally stimulated tactile feedback by a non-human primate in a reaching and grasping task.
- Developed new methods to discern motor intention in non-human primates.
- Determined the functional Magnetic Resonance Imaging (FMRI) signatures associated with expert status on DoD relevant tasks, which include skills that can make a direct translation to military benefit such as language acquisition, marksmanship, and threat detection.
- Commenced investigations into the neutral basis of expert performance using advanced functional neuroimaging technologies, state of the art spatio-temporal measurement techniques and novel signal processing methods.

FY 2008 Plans:
- Create an interface capable of enabling performance of a complex motor/sensory task through an assistive device.
- Map dynamic functional motor and sensory networks, develop methods for characterizing brain-wide sensory/motor tasks, and determine task performance changes resulting from learning and plasticity.
- Identify the specific brain networks and regions involved in the generation of expert performance; track and classify progression from novice to expert level using functional neuroimaging techniques.
- Investigate non-invasive interventions to increase the speed of expertise development and dramatically accelerate the transition from

novice to expert in key military tasks including neuropshyiologically-driven training regimens, neurally optimized stimuli, and stimulatory/modulatory interventions.

FY 2009 Plans:
- Develop prototype training systems to implement the acceleration methodologies for improved training.
- Explore the extrapolation of task specific acceleration techniques from limited domains to wider, more general training applications.
- Identify memory neural codes that are specific to critical work related tasks, enabling possible memory restoration in a brain-wounded warfighter.
- Leverage recent advances in neuroscience and mathematics to construct an integrated mathematical model of the brain that is consistent and predictive, rather than merely biologically inspired.
- Develop a theory that overcomes the difficulties present in traditional approaches, such as artificial intelligence and artificial neural network, to properly model complex human brain processes such as logical reasoning, language, mental computation, and context-dependent mental set.

check [Implant thoughts cause behavior—HAARP Program?

[Human-Assisted Neural Devices program

47

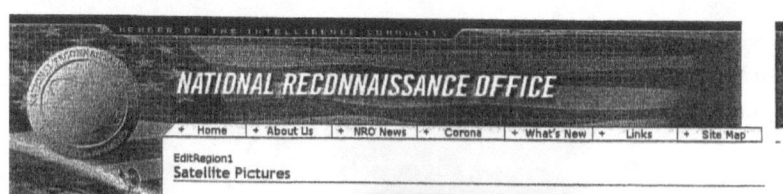

EditRegion1
Satellite Pictures

Sun, November 8, 2009

- Doing Business with the NRO
- How to Contact the NRO
- EEO Data for 'No Fear' Act
- The Freedom of Information Act
- The Office of Inspector General
- NRO and Operation Warfighter
- Technology Fellowship Program
- NROjr.gov - NRO's Kid's Page
- Site Policies

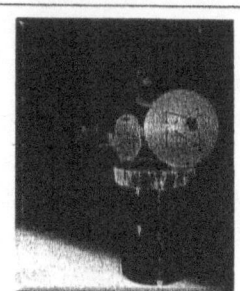

Above: An artist's rendition of a communications relay satellite.

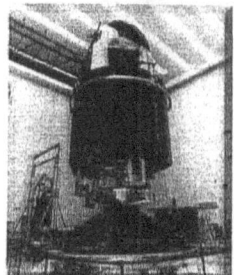

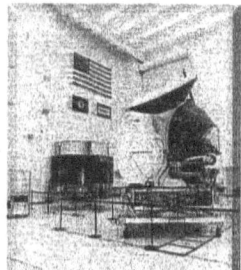

Above: Two views of a communications relay satellite.

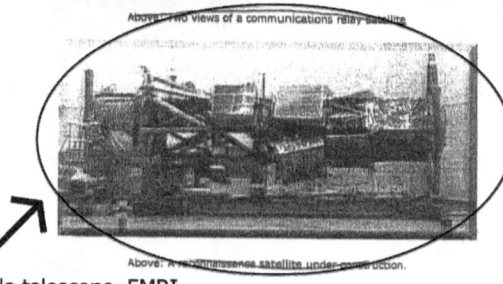

Above: A reconnaissance satellite under construction.

Picture the Hubble telescope, FMRI
technology; and infrared technology
focused on the earth, What do you get?

48

NSA, CIA, NRO EXHIBIT

I had to combine cases and requests for certain burdens placed on me (case no. 09-4281). The NSA refused to respond, violating FOIA guidelines. The CIA refused to process my request. The NRO said that they have no responsive records to my request. This is going to be a big lie one day. In the book *Spies, Lies and Whistleblowers*, the two ex-British agents claimed that files are held in two-stage retrievable method that if you ask for FMRI technology, you will need a code name and number to access FMRI technology. So they would not be lying by saying they could not locate any files, or they could make low-level no top secret searches and claim the same. This could be found on pages 115-116 in this book. Meanwhile, they are lying and conspiring to cover up actions.

US District Court
Eastern District of NY

Gilbert Roman, Plaintiff

V.   COMPLAINT

NSA, CIA, NRO, Defendants,

I request a Court ORDER ordering the complete search and release of all requested information

From the NSA, CIA, NRO. Exhibits A - $B3$ are from the NSA. Exhibits C - $C2$ are from the CIA.

Exhibits D - $D3$ are from the NRO. The court will see the NSA and CIA refuse to HONOR the

FREEDOM OF INFORMATION ACT.

Gilbert Roman
95-25-77th st
Ozone Pk., NY 11416

Gilbert R. Pro Se 10/1/09

REMEMBER TO RETURN 4 COMPLETE COPIES OF MY PAPER WORK: ALONG WITH THE RAISE SEAL

FROM THIS COURT IF YOU WANT ME TO SERVE ALL DEFENDANTS AND THE US ATTORNEYS OFFICE.

PEOPLE DO NOT REFUSE TO ANSWER IF THEY HAVE NOTHING TO HIDE.

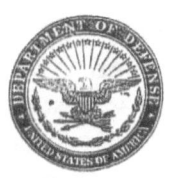

NATIONAL SECURITY AGENCY
CENTRAL SECURITY SERVICE

FORT GEORGE G. MEADE, MARYLAND 20755-6000

FOIA Case: 58310
1 April 2009

Mr. Gilbert Roman
95-25 77th Street
Ozone Park, NY 11416

This is the beginning of a
new book investigation!

Dear Mr. Roman:

This responds to your Freedom of Information Act (FOIA) request of 6 March 2009, which was received by this office on 11 March 2009, for information on functional magnetic resonance imaging, the date it was put into service, and the first successful report on the first person it was used on successfully.

For purposes of this request and based on the information you provided in your letter, you are considered an "all other" requester. As such, you are allowed 2 hours of search and the duplication of 100 pages at no cost. There are no assessable fees for this request.

The National Security Agency/Central Security Service (NSA/CSS) is the nation's cryptologic organization, and we have a twofold mission. Our Information Assurance mission is to provide solutions, products, and services to protect U.S. information infrastructures critical to national security interests. In response to requirements set at the highest levels of government, our Signals intelligence mission is to collect, process, and disseminate intelligence information from foreign signals for national foreign intelligence and counterintelligence purposes and to support military operations. Therefore, the information you request does not fall within the purview of this Agency, and a search for records responsive to your request would not be productive.

The fact that we have determined the subject of your request does not fall within the purview of this Agency may be considered by you as an adverse

51

determination. You are hereby advised of this Agency's appeal procedures. Any person notified of an adverse determination may file an appeal to the NSA/CSS Freedom of Information Act Appeal Authority. The appeal must be postmarked no later than 60 calendar days after the date of the initial denial letter. The appeal shall be in writing addressed to the NSA/CSS FOIA Appeal Authority (DJP4), National Security Agency, 9800 Savage Road STE 6248, Fort George G. Meade, MD 20755-6248. To aid in processing the appeal, it should reference the adverse determination and explain in sufficient detail and particularity the grounds upon which you believe a search is warranted. The NSA/CSS FOIA Appeal Authority will endeavor to respond to the appeal within 20 working days after receipt, absent unusual circumstances.

We have enclosed a fact sheet describing NSA/CSS's mission, which we hope you will find useful and informative.

Sincerely,

PAMELA N. PHILLIPS
Acting Initial Denial Authority

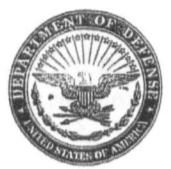

NATIONAL SECURITY AGENCY
CENTRAL SECURITY SERVICE

FORT GEORGE G. MEADE, MARYLAND 20755-6000

FOIA Case: 59231
5 August 2009

Mr. Gilbert Roman   The beginning of new
95-25 77th Street   book research.
Ozone Park, NY 11416

Dear Mr. Roman:

This responds to your Freedom of Information Act (FOIA) request of 18 July 2009, which was received by this office on 23 July 2009, for the following:

1. Information on the technology that allows you to send thoughts or implant thought to the person you are focused on;
2. The day it was perfected; the report on the first person it was used against successfully;
3. The report on how you can also cause behavior with this technology;
4. A complete search of all records from top secret to lowest level, to include stored and vaulted micro-film or documents records;
5. This information could be under HAARP systems but as you know you could hide records under any name and get a no records response.

Your request has been assigned Case Number 59231.

Please be advised that this Agency is in receipt of your FOIA request received 11 March 2009 for records on magnetic resonance imaging, the date it was put into service, and the first successful report on the first person it was used on successfully. For that request (FOIA Case 58310), we responded to you that the subject of your request was not within the purview of this Agency. We interpret this current request from you to be on the same or similar topic, and our response remains the same: the subject of this request is not within the purview of the National Security Agency. For your convenience, we have enclosed a copy of your previous request and our response letter dated 1 April 2009.

[They refuse to process my request!]

Because this Agency has already responded to you on this topic and has fully complied with its FOIA obligation, any future requests made by you concerning this topic will be filed with your previous FOIA case with no further action by this Agency.

Sincerely,

Marianne Stupar

PAMELA N. PHILLIPS
Chief
FOIA/PA Office

Encls:
a/s

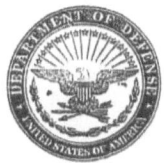

NATIONAL SECURITY AGENCY

FORT GEORGE G. MEADE, MARYLAND 20755-6000

Case No. 58310/Appeal No. 3435
11 September 2009

Mr. Gilbert Roman
95-25 77th Street
Ozone Park, NY 11416

Dear Mr. Roman:

I am writing in response to your letter, postmarked 8 April 2008, appealing the National Security Agency's (NSA) determination that your Freedom of Information Act (FOIA) request fails to fall within the purview of this Agency. You had requested "information on Functional magnetic resonance imaging; the date it was put into service; and the first successful report on the first person it was used on successfully." I have reviewed your original request, the Acting Initial Denial Authority's response to you, and your letter of appeal. Based on my review, I have determined that requests for information concerning the records described above do not relate to NSA's two-fold mission, which was explained in the Acting Initial Denial Authority's letter to you, dated 1 April 2009. Therefore, the information you requested does not fall within the purview of this Agency, and a search for records responsive to your request would not be product.

It is my understanding that you have already filed a lawsuit against the Agency in the United States District Court for the Eastern District of New York. My records indicate that you filed said lawsuit on or about 15 July 2009 seeking judicial review of NSA's Acting Initial Denial Authority's denial of your 6 March 2009 request under the FOIA. I understand that this lawsuit was filed while your 8 April 2009 appeal was pending before the FOIA/PA Appeals Authority. Nevertheless, since I am denying your appeal herein, in accordance with 5 U.S.C. § 552(a)(6)(A)(ii), you are hereby advised of your right to seek judicial review of my decision in the United States District Court in the district in which you reside, in which you have your principal place of business, in which the Agency records are situated (United States District Court of Maryland), or in the District of Columbia.

Sincerely,

JOHN C. INGLIS
Freedom of Information Act/Privacy Act
Appeals Authority

Gilbert Roman
95-25 77th St
Ozone pk., NY 11416
July 18, 2009

This request is made under the FREEDOM of Information Act and/or Privacy Act of 1974. My request is as follows:

1. Information on the technology that allows you to send thoughts or implant thoughts to the person you are focused on.
2. The day it was perfected; the report on the first person it was used against successfully.
3. The report on how you can also cause behavior; with this technology,
4. A complete search of all records from top secret to lowest level; to include stored and vaulted micro-film or documents records.
5. This information could be under W.A.R.P. systems but as you know you could hide records under any name and get a no records response.

This request should be made free of charge because of the civil rights violation, constitutional violations, against the AMERICAN people. If you can not make it free of charge I will authorize to pay 100 dollars a month for searches; when cleared by me. Do not lie. Cover-up the truth because there will be judicial review and soon uninterrupted media coverage. The truth will set you free.

Thank You.

Gilbert Roman
95-25 77th St.
Ozone Pk., NY 11416
Aug. 10, 2009

Re: FOIA case 59231

This is an appeal of your denial to process my request. Attached you shall find my request and your response not to make searches. This request should be made free of charge because of the public interest. Also because of all the civil and constitutional violations of the mis-use of modern day technology and none application of modern day technology. If you can not make my request free of charge I will authorize to pay 100 dollars a month; upon my approval.

Central Intelligence Agency

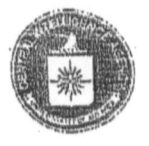

Washington, D.C. 20505

July 30, 2009

Mr. Gilbert Roman   Tru TV broadcast December 3, 2009,
95-25 77th St   in *Conspiracy Theory with Jesse*
Ozone Park, NY 11416   *Ventura*—HAARP program

Reference: F-2009-01444

Dear Mr. Roman:

This is a final response to your 18 July 2009 Freedom of Information Act (FOIA) request, received in the office of the Information and Privacy Coordinator on 24 July 2009, for records on the following:

1. Information on the technology that allows you to send thoughts or implant thoughts to the person you are focused on.
2. The day it was perfected; the report on the first person it was used against successfully.
3. The report on how you can also cause behavior; with this technology.
4. A complete search of all records from top secret to lowest level; to include stored and vaulted micro-film or documents records.
5. This information could be under HAARP systems but as you know you could hide records under any name and get a no records response.
6. Information on functional Magnetic Resonance Imaging FMRI.
7. The date it was put into service.
8. The report on the first person it was used against successfully.
9. A complete search of all records from top-secret to lowest level; to include stored and vaulted micro-film and documents.
10. An affidavit signed to state the degree of top-secret or lower level searches were made. To include how many minutes or hours searches were made.

Your FOIA request cannot be accepted in its current form, because it would require the agency to perform an unreasonably burdensome search. The FOIA requires requesters to "reasonably describe" the information they seek so that professional employees familiar with the subject matter can locate responsive information with a reasonable amount of effort. Because of the breadth and lack of specificity of your request, and the way in which our records systems are configured, the Agency cannot conduct a reasonable search for information responsive to your request. We encourage you to refine the scope of your request (such as including a time frame for, and narrower, more specific descriptions of, the information you seek) to enable us to conduct a reasonable search for responsive information.

Sincerely,

Delores M. Nelson
Information and Privacy Coordinator

Gilbert Roman
95-25 77th st.
Ozone pk., NY 11416
Aug. 6, 2009

Re: F-2009-01444

    This is an appeal of your denial to process my request. Attached you shall find my request and your response. I stated that this request should be made free of charge because of the civil rights violations, constitutional violations against the American people. If they could not be made free of I will authorize to pay 100 dollars a month for services; when cleared by me. Not to search is in direct violation of the Freedom of Information Act and/or Privacy Act of 1974. So yet another court case will take place if you still refuse to uphold and defend the constitution of the US on foreign and domestic soil; from all who would violate it.

Gilbert Roman
95-25 77th st
Ozone pk., NY 11416
July 18, 2009

This request is made under the FREEDOM of Information Act and/or Privacy Act of 1974. My request is as follows:

1. Information on the technology that allows you to send thoughts or implant thoughts to the person you are focused on.
2. The day it was perfected; the report on the first person it was used against successfully.
3. The report on how you can also cause behavior; with this technology,
4. A complete search of all records from top secret to lowest level; to include stored and vaulted micro-film or documents records.
5. This information could be under W.A.R.P. systems but as you know you could hide records under any name and get a no records response.
6. Information on Fractional Magnetic Resonance Imaging FMRI.
7. The date it was put into service.
8. The report on the first person it was used against successfully.
9. A complete search of all records from top-secret to lowest level; to include stored and vaulted micro-film and documents.
10. An affidavit signed to state the degree of top-secret or lower level searches were made. To include how many minutes or hours searches were made. This request should be made free of charge because of the civil rights violation, constitutional violations, against the AMERICAN people. If you can not make it free of charge I will authorize to pay 100 dollars a month for searches; when cleared by me. Do not lie. Cover-up the truth because there will be judicial review and soon uninterrupted media coverage. The truth will set you free.

Thank You.

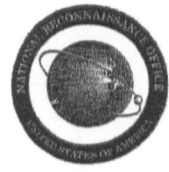

NATIONAL RECONNAISSANCE OFFICE

14675 Lee Road
Chantilly, VA 20151-1715

23 July 2009

Gilbert Roman
95-25 77th Street
Ozone Park, NY 11416

Dear Mr. Roman:

This is in response to your letter, dated 18 July 2009, received in the Information Management Services Center of the National Reconnaissance Office (NRO) on 23 July 2009. Pursuant to the Freedom of Information Act (FOIA), you are requesting:

"1. . . . Information on the technology that allows you to send thoughts or implant thoughts to the person you are focused on.
2. The day it was perfected; the report on the first person it was used against successfully.
3. The report on how you can also cause behavior; with this technology."

We have accepted your request. It will be processed in accordance with the FOIA, 5 U.S.C. § 552, as amended, and the NRO Operational File Exemption, 50 U.S.C. § 432a. Unless you object, we will limit our search to NRO-originated records existing through the date of this acceptance letter.

Since we may not respond within the 20 working days stipulated by the Act, you have the right to consider this as a denial and may appeal to the NRO Appeal Review Panel. It would seem more reasonable, however, to have us continue processing your request and respond as soon as we can. You may appeal any denial of records at that time. Unless we hear from you otherwise, we will assume that you agree, and will proceed on this basis. Fees are incurred whether we find responsive records or not.

The FOIA authorizes federal agencies to assess fees for record services. Based upon the information provided, you have been placed in the "other" category of requesters, which means you are responsible for the cost of search time exceeding two hours ($44.00/hour) and reproduction fees (.15 per page) exceeding 100 pages.

In your letter, you indicated a willingness "to pay 100 dollars a month for searches; when cleared by me." We will notify you if assessable fees meet or exceed our minimum billing threshold of $25.00.

Regarding your request for a few waiver, please be advised that fee waivers or reductions are granted when there is a public interest in disclosure of information, which will contribute significantly to the public's understanding of the operations or activities of the NRO. A decision to waive or reduce fees cannot be made until after any responsive documents to be disclosed have been reviewed for "public interest".

If you have any questions, please call the Requester Service Center at (703) 227-9326 and reference case number F09-0108.

Sincerely,

Linda S. Hathaway
Chief, Information Access
and Release Team

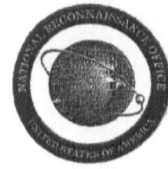

NATIONAL RECONNAISSANCE OFFICE
14675 Lee Road
Chantilly, VA 20151-1715

19 August 2009

Gilbert Roman
95-25 77th Street
Ozone Park, NY 11416

Dear Mr. Roman:

This is in response to your letter, dated 18 July 2009, received in the Information Management Services Center of the National Reconnaissance Office (NRO) on 23 July 2009. Pursuant to the Freedom of Information Act (FOIA), you are requesting:

"1. . . . Information on the technology that allows you to send thoughts or implant thoughts to the person you are focused on.
2. The day it was perfected; the report on the first person it was used against successfully.
3. The report on how you can also cause behavior; with this technology."

Your request was processed in accordance with the FOIA, 5 U.S.C. § 552, as amended, and the NRO Operational File Exemption, 50 U.S.C. § 432a. A thorough search for NRO-originated records in our files and databases revealed that we have no responsive records pertaining to your request.

The FOIA authorizes federal agencies to assess fees for record services. Based upon the information provided, you have been placed in the "other" category of requesters, which means you are responsible for the cost of search time exceeding two hours ($44.00/hour) and reproduction fees (.15 per page) exceeding 100 pages. Fees incurred in processing your request are $22.00 for ½ hour search time in excess of the two hours provided at no charge under the FOIA. As this amount is less than our $25.00 billing threshold, these fees are being waived.

You have the right to appeal this determination by addressing your appeal to the NRO Appeal Authority, 14675 Lee Road, Chantilly, VA 20151-1715, within 60 days of the date of this letter. Should you decide to do so, please explain the basis of your appeal.

If you have any questions, please all the Requester Service Center at (703) 227-9326 and reference case number F09-0108.

Sincerely,

Linda S. Hathaway
Chief, Information Access
and Release Team

Gilbert Roman
95-25 77th st
Ozone pk., NY 11416
July 18, 2009

This request is made under the FREEDOM of Information Act and/or Privacy Act of 1974. My request is as follows:

1. Information on the technology that allows you to send thoughts or implant thoughts to the person you are focused on.
2. The day it was perfected; the report on the first person it was used against successfully.
3. The report on how you can also cause behavior; with this technology,
4. A complete search of all records from top secret to lowest level; to include stored and vaulted micro-film or documents records.
5. This information could be under W.A.R.P. systems but as you know you could hide records under any name and get a no records response.

This request should be made free of charge because of the civil rights violation, constitutional violations, against the AMERICAN people. If you can not make it free of charge I will authorize to pay 100 dollars a month for searches; when cleared by me. Do not lie. Cover-up the truth because there will be judicial review and soon uninterrupted media coverage. The truth will set you free.

Thank You.

Gilbert Roman
95-25 77th st
Ozone Pk., NY 11416
Sept. 3, 2009

Re: NRO APPEAL F09-0108

    This is an appeal of your response letter dated Aug. 19, 2009. I respectfully request that further searches be made. From top secret to lower level searches. And remember the name of the system may be W.A.R.P. systems. That this request should be made free of charge because of the public interest. If you can not make it free of charge; please bill me for your cost. Attached you shall find all request and responses.

Respectfully Submitted,

_____

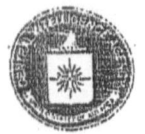

2 December 2009

Mr. Gilbert Roman
95-25 77th Street
Ozone Park, NY 11416

Reference: F-2009-00753

Dear Mr. Roman:

This is further to our 11 June 2009 response to your 6 March 2009 Freedom of Information Act (FOIA) request for "all copies of the Freedom of Information Processing forms used on all of my request [sic] to your agency over the years."

During a review of your request, we discovered that our response inadvertently failed to address eight documents responsive to your request. Enclosed are two documents that can be released in a segregable form with deletions made on the basis of FOIA exemptions (b)(3) and (b)(5). The six remaining documents must be denied in their entirety on the basis of FOIA exemptions (b)(3) and (b)(5). An explanation of exemptions is enclosed. As the CIA Information and Privacy Coordinator, I am the Agency official responsible for these determinations. Because the information in question is the subject of pending litigation in federal court, the CIA cannot accept any administrative appeal of these determinations, in accordance with 32 C.F.R. § 1900.42(c).

Sincerely,

Delores M. Nelson
Information and Privacy Coordinator

Enclosures

C05462127

ADMINISTRATIVE INTERNAL USE ONLY
PIRD MEMO
F-1999-00952

DATE: 05/08/2000

MEMO TO: IRG DATABASE

FROM: William H. McNair
           DO Information Review Officer

SUBJECT:

Case Number: F-1999-00952 OPENI
Tasked on: 11/03/99
Requester: ROMAN , GILBERT
Case Subject: 1. COPIES OF FORMS USED IN PROCESSING FOIA
REQUESTS
2. SATELLITE RECORDS OF A PERSON IN WOODBRIDGE, NJ. AND
OGDENSBURG, NY

REPLY:

C05462128

(b) (3)
(b) (5)

PIRD MEMO
F-1999-00952

DATE: 11/08/99

MEMO TO: IRG DATABASE

FROM: _____

Associate Information Review Officer, DDA

SUBJECT: Case Number: F-1999-00952 OPENI
               Tasked on: 06/10/99
               Requester: ROMAN , GILBERT
               Case Subject: 1. COPIES OF FORMS USED IN PROCESSING
               FOIA REQUESTS
               2. SATELLITE RECORDS OF A PERSON IN WOODBRIDGE,
               NJ. AND OGDENSBURG, NY

REPLY:

    1. This is in response to Gilbert Roman's 21 April 1999 FOIA request for
"copies of the forms used to process all of [his] FOIA and/or PA requests to [our]
agency." Our processing included a search for records in existence as of and
through the date of the acceptance letter, 10 June 1999, in accordance with the
FOIA and the CIA Information Act.

    2. The Directorate of Administration (DA) conducted a search for records
as specified above and located documents responsive to Mr. Roman's request.

    3. A paper copy of this response is forthcoming. Meanwhile, this
concludes DA's action on this request.

Attachments

NO RECORD FOUND	☐ YES
RELEASED IN FULL	
DENIED IN PART	
DENIED IN FULL	
INTERNAL COORD	

APPROVED FOR RELEASE☐
DATE: 01-Dec-2009

INTERNAL REFERRAL	
EXTERNAL COORD	
EXTERNAL REFERRAL	

Sent on: 11/08/99

Explanation of Exemptions

Freedom of Information Act:

(b)(1)   exempts from disclosure information currently and properly classified, pursuant to an Executive Order;

(b)(2)   exempts from disclosure information, which pertains solely to the internal personnel rules and practices of the Agency;

(b)(3)   exempts from disclosure information that another federal statute protects, provided that the other federal statute either requires that the matters be withheld, or establishes particular criteria for withholding or refers to particular types of matters to be withheld. The (b)(3) statutes upon which the CIA relies include, but are not limited to, the CIA Act of 1949;

(b)(4)   exempts from disclosure trade secrets and commercial or financial information that is obtained from a person and that is privileged or confidential;

(b)(5)   exempts from disclosure inter—and intra-agency memoranda or letters that would not be available by law to a party other than an agency in litigation with the agency;

(b)(6)   exempts from disclosure information from personnel and medical files and similar files the disclosure of which would constitute a clearly unwarranted invasion of privacy;

(b)(7)   exempts from disclosure information compiled for law enforcement purposes to the extent that the production of the information (A) could reasonably be expected to interfere with enforcement proceedings; (B) would deprive a person of a right to a fair trial or an impartial adjudication; (C) could reasonably be expected to constitute an unwarranted invasion of personal privacy; (D) could reasonably be expected to disclose the identity of a confidential source or, in the case of information compiled by a criminal law enforcement authority in the course of a criminal investigation or by an agency conducting a lawful national security intelligence investigation, information furnished by a confidential source; (E) would disclose techniques and procedures for law enforcement investigations or prosecutions if such disclosure could reasonably be expected to risk circumvention of the law; or (F) could reasonably be expected to endanger any individual's life or physical safety;

(b)(8) exempts from disclosure information contained in reports or related to examination, operating, or condition reports prepared by, or on behalf of, or for use of an agency responsible for regulating or supervising financial institutions; and

(b)(9) exempts from disclosure geological and geophysical information and data, including maps, concerning wells.

January 2007

ANOTHER CASE AGAINST THE CIA, CASE NO. 09-3344

This case is also in the Eastern District of New York; ask for documents used to process my FOIA request to the CIA over the years. I received sixteen documents. I was sent a page that was not clear, and no page showed search time for searches. How could searches be made with no search time entered? I also showed FOIA forms from the NRO and NASA, which showed no search time entered and only low-level searches made. Were searches ever made? Are they lying in my response letters? These and many other questions need to be answered. On one of the forms released, someone wrote, "I plan not to respond." What did he mean by this?

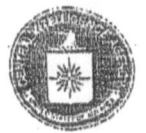

June 11, 2009

Mr. Gilbert Roman
95-25 77th Street
Ozone Park, NY 11416

Reference: F-2009-00753

Dear Mr. Roman:

This is a final response to your 6 March 2009 Freedom of Information Act (FOIA) request for "all copies of the Freedom of Information Processing forms used on all of my request [sic] to your agency over the years." We processed your request in accordance with the FOIA, 5 U.S.C. § 552, as amended, and the CIA Information Act, 50 U.S.C. § 431, as amended. Our processing included a re-review of the denied information in the documents previously released to you in F-1999-00952 that were responsive to this request

Enclosed are 14 documents responsive to your request which can be released in segregable form with deletions made on the basis of FOIA exemptions (b)(3). An explanation of exemptions is enclosed. You may appeal my decision to the Agency Release Panel, in my care, within 45 days from the date of this letter. Please include the basis of your appeal.

Sincerely,

Delores M. Nelson
Information and Privacy Coordinator

Enclosures

75

Explanation of Exemptions

Freedom of Information Act:

(b)(1) exempts from disclosure information currently and properly classified, pursuant to an Executive Order;

(b)(2) exempts from disclosure information, which pertains solely to the internal personnel rules and practices of the Agency;

(b)(3) exempts from disclosure information that another federal statute protects, provided that the other federal statute either requires that the matters be withheld, or establishes particular criteria for withholding or refers to particular types of matters to be withheld. The (b)(3) statutes upon which the CIA relies include, but are not limited to, the CIA Act of 1949;

(b)(4) exempts from disclosure trade secrets and commercial or financial information that is obtained from a person and that is privileged or confidential;

(b)(5) exempts from disclosure inter- and intra-agency memoranda or letters that would not be available by law to a party other than an agency in litigation with the agency;

(b)(6) exempts from disclosure information from personnel and medical files and similar files the disclosure of which would constitute a clearly unwarranted invasion of privacy;

(b)(7) exempts from disclosure information compiled for law enforcement purposes to the extent that the production of the information (A) could reasonably be expected to interfere with enforcement proceedings; (B) would deprive a person of a right to a fair trial or an impartial adjudication; (C) could reasonably be expected to constitute an unwarranted invasion of personal privacy; (D) could reasonably be expected to disclose the identity of a confidential source or, in the case of information compiled by a criminal law enforcement authority in the course of a criminal investigation or by an agency conducting a lawful national security intelligence investigation, information furnished by a confidential source; (E) would disclose techniques and procedures for law enforcement investigations or prosecutions if such disclosure could reasonably be expected to risk circumvention of the law; or (F) could reasonably be expected to endanger any individual's life or physical safety;

(b)(8)   exempts from disclosure information contained in reports or related to examination, operating, or condition reports prepared by, or on behalf of, or for use of an agency responsible for regulating or supervising financial institutions; and

(b)(9)   exempts from disclosure geological and geophysical information and data, including maps, concerning wells.

January 2007

(b) (3)

PRIVACY ACT REQUEST

SUBJECT: (Optional) RE: INFO ON SELF				REQUEST NUMBER	
ROMAN, GILBERT				P96-1518	

FROM:		EXTENSION	DATE SENT		
IP&CRD/MSG/OIT			5 August 1996		
			SUSPENSE DATE		

TO: (Officer designation, room number, and building)	DATE		OFFICER'S INITIALS	COMMENTS (Number each comment to show from whom to whom. Draw a line across column after each comment.)
	RECEIVED	FORWARDED		
1. DDA/IRO-Mr.Hatch 1236 Ames Bldg.				Please process the attached Privacy request.
2.				PLEASE PROCESS UNDER PA & FOIA
3.				SEARCH CUT OFF DATE: 30 July 96
4. RETURN TO: DDA/IRO-Mr.Hatch 1236 Ames Bldg.				FEE CATEGORY: No Fees
5.				PLS NOTE: CR: F96-0018
6. DDO/				
7.				
8.				
9.				
10.				
11.				ACTION: DDA/IRO, DDO/IRO
12.				INFO: DDA/IRO

APPROVED FOR RELEASED
DATE: 10-Jun-2009

RETURN TO:
IP&CRD/MSG/OIT 1107 Ames Bldg. -

PRIVACY ACT REQUEST

FORM 3834 OBSOLETE PREVIOUS
12-79 EDITIONS

78

DA (b)(3)

PRIVACY ACT REQUEST

SUBJECT: (Optional) RE: INFO ON SELF					REQUEST NUMBER	
ROMAN, GILBERT					P96-1518	

FROM:			EXTENSION	DATE SENT 5 August 1996	
IP&CRD/MSG/OIT				SUSPENSE DATE	

TO: (Officer designation, room number, and building)	DATE		OFFICER'S INITIALS	COMMENTS (Number each comment to show from whom to whom. Draw a line across column after each comment.)
	RECEIVED	FORWARDED		
1. DDA/IRO-Mr.Hatch 1236 Ames Bldg.				Please process the attached Privacy request.
2.				PLEASE PROCESS UNDER PA & FOIA
3.				SEARCH CUT OFF DATE: 30 July 96
4. RETURN TO: DDA/IRO-Mr.Hatch 1236 Ames Bldg.				FEE CATEGORY: No Fees
5.				PLS NOTE: CR: F96-8018
6. DDO/	13 Aug. 96			NOT clear
7.				Subject has been searched with all ... ... accounts of this Directorate which ... do have an interest or record. This ... ... ctorate has no information which ... ... be identified with ...
8.				
9.				... Directorate of Operations 13 Sep 76
10.				ACTION: DDA/IRO, DDO/IRO
11.				INFO: DDA/IRO
12.				APPROVED FOR RELEASED DATE: 10-Jun-2009

RETURN TO:
IP&CRD/MSG/OIT 1107 Ames Bldg.

Sep 11 11:00 AM '96

PRIVACY ACT REQUEST

NO time entered for searches?

C05390974

(b) (3)

CASE: F97-0891 FROM: [   ] DATE: 4/15/97

[ ] New Request
[ ] Other agency referral and/or coordination
[ ] Other agency referral and/or coordination in appeal
ACTION REQUIRED:

[ ] Prepare Freedom Form letter #2 (return to Case Officer
 after mailing and logging)
Case Officer Initials:____
[ ] Prepare Privacy Form Letter: [ ]#1 [ ]#2 [ ]#3 [ ]#4
[ ] Enter subject change (see att.)   Logging initials:____
[ ] Enter the following keywords (20 characters per keyword):

_____   _____
_____   _____
_____   Logging initials:____
                                     Date:_____

                [ ]ORIS/MORI:

[ ] [   ] search ORIS for all records regarding _____
                                                  _____
[ ] [   ] search MORI for all records regarding _____
            not located as a result of the ORIS search

NOTE:[ ] Provide documents
[ ] Provide Case Officer & Requester printouts

 If Case Officer is aware of any particular cases under which
documents desired may have [   ] been released within the last two
years, please advise [   ] and [   ] of this fact. The reason
that this information would be useful to [   ] and [   ] is
due to ORIS' two-year indexing backlog of material released
during that timeframe.

[ ] Material on _____ was
    released under Case No.(s)_____.

                [ ] IA Tasking:

[ ] Fees Category: Commercial Educational/Scientific
                    U.S. News Media   All Other

[ ] Request processing under FOIA/PA (Circle if applicable)
[ ] Circle and/or list additional components:

    DA   DCI   DI   DO   DST

SUBJECT BLOCK: _____
              _____

ROUTE SLIP.TXT

C05390975

(b)(3)

CASE: F97-0522 FROM [   ] DATE: 2/24/97

[ ] New Request
[ ] Other agency referral and/or coordination
[ ] Other agency referral and/or coordination in appeal
                ACTION REQUIRED:

[ ] Prepare Freedom Form letter #2 (return to Case Officer
 after mailing and logging)
Case Officer Initials: ____
[ ] Prepare Privacy Form Letter: [ ]#1 [ ]#2 [ ]#3 [ ]#4
[ ] Enter subject change (see att.)   Logging initials: ____
[✓] Enter the following keywords (20 characters per keyword):
_____
_____   Logging initials: [   ]
                                                  Date: 3/26/97
                [ ]ORIS/MORI:

[ ] [   ] search ORIS for all records regarding _____

[ ] [   ] search MORI for all records regarding _____
               not located as a result of the ORIS search

NOTE:[ ] Provide documents
[ ] Provide Case Officer & Requester printouts

  If Case Officer is aware of any particular cases under which
documents desired may have been released within the last two
years, please advise [   ] and [   ] of this fact. The reason
that this information would be useful to [   ] and [ ] is
due to ORIS' two-year indexing backlog of material released
during that timeframe.

[ ] Material on _____ was
    released under Case No.(s) _____.

                [ ] IA Tasking:

[ ] Fees Category: Commercial Educational/Scientific
                    U.S. News Media   All Other

[ ] Request processing under FOIA/PA (Circle if applicable)
[ ] Circle and/or list additional components:

      DA   DCI   DI   DO   DST

SUBJECT BLOCK: _____
_____
ROUTE SLIP.TXT

APPROVED FOR RELEASED
DATE: 10-Jun-2009

SLIP.TXT

CASE: *F96 - 2158* FROM: [   ] DATE: *12/18/96*

[ ] New Request
[ ] Other agency referral and/or coordination
[ ] Other agency referral and/or coordination in appeal
              ACTION REQUIRED:

[ ] Prepare Freedom Form letter #2 (return to Case Officer
 after mailing and logging)
Case Officer Initials:____
[ ] Prepare Privacy Form Letter: [ ]#1 [ ]#2 [ ]#3 [ ]#4
[ ] Enter subject change (see att.)   Logging initials:____
[ ] Enter the following keywords (20 characters per keyword):
                                        scientist
satellites in orbit   *medical doctor*
abst   Logging initials:____
                                        Date: *12/19/96*
              [ ]ORIS/MORI:

[ ] [   ]   search ORIS for all records regarding _____
                 _____
[ ] [   ]   search MORI for all records regarding _____
        [   ] not located as a result of the ORIS search

NOTE:[ ] Provide documents
[ ] Provide Case Officer & Requester printouts

 If Case Officer is aware of any particular cases under which
documents desired may have been released within the last two
years, please advise [   ] and [   ] of this fact. The reason
that this information would be useful to [   ] and [   ] is
due to ORIS' two-year indexing backlog of material released
during that timeframe.

[ ] Material on _____ was
    released under Case No.(s) _____ .

              [ ] IA Tasking:

[ ] Fees Category: Commercial Educational/Scientific
                    U.S. News Media   All Other

[ ] Request processing under FOIA/PA (Circle if applicable)
[ ] Circle and/or list additional components:

    DA   DCI   DI   DO   DST

SUBJECT BLOCK:_____

ROUTE SLIP.TXT _____

C05390977

(b)(3)

CASE: *F96-0018*   FROM: [   ]   DATE: _1/2/96_

[X] New Request
[ ] Other agency referral and/or coordination
[ ] Other agency referral and/or coordination in appeal

ACTION REQUIRED:

[ ] Prepare Freedom Form letter #2   (return to Case Officer
    after mailing and logging)   Case Officer Initials:____
[ ] Prepare Privacy Form Letter: [ ]#1 [ ]#2 [ ]#3 [ ]#4
[ ] Enter subject change (see att.)   Logging initials:____
[ ] Enter the following keywords (20 characters per keyword):
                                        device
_____   *pulses & human brain*
Agency leaders   *patterns of hu___ brain*
names and addresses   Logging initials [ ]
                                                  V& *-96*

[ ]ORIS/MORI:

[ ] [   ] search ORIS for all records regarding _____

[ ] [   ] search MORI for all records regarding _____
    _____ not located as a result of the ORIS search

NOTE: [ ] Provide documents
         [ ] Provide Case Officer & Requester printouts

     If Case Officer is aware of any particular cases under
which documents desired may have been released within the
last two years, please advise[   ]and[   ]of this fact.
The reason that this information would be useful to[   ]and
[   ]is due to ORIS' two-year indexing backlog of material
released during that timeframe.

[ ] Material on _____ was
    released under Case No.(s)_____.

              [ ] IA Tasking:

[ ] Fees Category: Commercial   Educational/Scientific
                    U.S. News Media   All Other
[ ] Request processing under FOIA/PA (Circle if applicable)
[ ] Circle and/or list additional components:
         DO   DI   DA   DS&T   DCI

SUBJECT BLOCK: _____

_____

_____

GENERAL [   ]

C05390978

(b) (3)

CASE: *F97-0155* FROM: [____] DATE: __3/___97__

[ ] New Request
[ ] Other agency referral and/or coordination
[ ] Other agency referral and/or coordination in appeal
ACTION REQUIRED:

[ ] Prepare Freedom Form letter #2 (return to Case Officer
after mailing and logging)
Case Officer Initials:____
[ ] Prepare Privacy Form Letter: [ ]#1 [ ]#2 [ ]#3 [ ]#4
[ ] Enter subject change (see att.) Logging initials:____
[✓] Enter the following keywords (20 characters per keyword):

remote viewing

Logging initials: [____]
Date: _4/11/97_

[ ]ORIS/MORI:

[ ] [____] search ORIS for all records regarding _____

[ ] [____] search MORI for all records regarding _____
_____ not located as a result of the ORIS search

NOTE:[ ] Provide documents
[ ] Provide Case Officer & Requester printouts

If Case Officer is aware of any particular cases under which
documents desired may have been released within the last two
years, please advise [____] and [____] of this fact. The reason
that this information would be useful to [____] and [____] is
due to ORIS' two-year indexing backlog of material released
during that timeframe.

[ ] Material on _____ was
released under Case No.(s)_____.

[ ] IA Tasking:

[ ] Fees Category: Commercial Educational/Scientific
U.S. News Media All Other

[ ] Request processing under FOIA/PA (Circle if applicable)
[ ] Circle and/or list additional components:

DA DCI DI DO DST

SUBJECT BLOCK:_____

ROUTE SLIP.TXT

no tasking

APPROVED FOR RELEASE□
DATE: 10-Jun-2009

84

C05390979

(b)(3)

CASE: P 96-1518 FROM [   ]   DATE: 7/29/1996

[x] New Request
[ ] Other agency referral and/or coordination
[ ] Other agency referral and/or coordination in appeal

ACTION REQUIRED:

[ ] Prepare Freedom Form letter #2   (return to Case Officer
      after mailing and logging)   Case Officer Initials:___
[ ] Prepare Privacy Form Letter: [ ]#1 [ ]#2 [ ]#3 [ ]#4
[ ] Enter subject change (see att.)   Logging initials:___
[ ] Enter the following keywords (20 characters per keyword):

_____   _____

_____   _____

_____   Logging initials:___

                    [ ]ORIS/MORI:

[[   ] : search ORIS for all records regarding _____

[[   ]   search MORI for all records regarding _____
   _____ not located as a result of the ORIS search

NOTE: [ ] Provide documents
           [ ] Provide Case Officer & Requester printouts

       If Case Officer is aware of any particular cases under
which documents desired may have been released within the
last two years, please advise[   ]and[   ]of this fact.
The reason that this information would be useful to[   ]and
[   ]is due to ORIS' two-year indexing backlog of material
released during that timeframe.

[*] Material on _____ was
      released under Case No.(s)_____.

                    [X] IA Tasking:

[ ] Fees Category: Commercial 1   Educational/Scientific 2
                     U.S. News Media 3 All Other 4
[ ] Request processing under FOIA/PA (Circle if applicable)
[ ] Circle and/or list additional components:
     (DA)   DCI   DI   (DO)   DS&T
SUBJECT BLOCK:
   Mr. Gilbert. for information on self

GENERAL [   ]

APPROVED FOR RELEASE☐
DATE: 10-Jun-2009

C05390980

SECURE FACSIMILE TRANSMITTAL FORM

DATE: **7-29-96**

SENDING SECURE/FAX TELEPHONE NUMBER:

RECEIVING SECURE/FAX TELEPHONE NUMBER

NUMBER OF PAGES (Including Transmittal Form and Coversheet, if applicable) 26

FROM:

(Name / Office / Extension)

SUBJECT:

TO: (ADDRESSEE / ORGANIZATION / OFFICE / EXTENSION)

1.	
2.	
3.	
4.	
5.	
6.	
7.	
8.	
9.	
10.	

SPECIAL INSTRUCTIONS:

RELEASING OFFICIAL:

(PRINTED NAME)   (SIGNATURE)

RECEIVING STATION USE ONLY

Please receipt for material by entering time of receipt/signature and transmit back to sending station.

DATE / TIME: SIGNATURE:

APPROVED FOR RELEASED
DATE: 10-Jun-2009

FORM
10-92   4383A   (EF)   (CLASSIFICATION OF MATERIAL TRANSMITTED)

86

(b) (3)

IRRG TASKING TO THE DIRECTORATE IRO

Distribution:

DIRECTORATE	ADDRESS	TASK DATE
DA		06/10/99

CASE NUMBER: F-1999-00952   TASKED: 06/10/99

External Case Info: External Source: Ext Agency: External Due Date:
      SEARCH
      External Number:

REQUESTER: ROMAN , GILBERT   POC:

SUBJECT: 1. COPIES OF FORMS USED IN PROCESSING FOIA REQUESTS

2. SATELLITE RECORDS OF A PERSON IN WOODBRIDGE, N.J. AND

OGDENSBURG, NY

COORD FROM:		REFER FROM:	
All DIRs TASKED:	DA	DIR TASKED:	DA
DOC COUNT:	0	CR:	
FEE CATEGORY	NONE	CASE STATUS:	OPENI
CASE OFFICER:		PHONE:	
IA:		PHONE:	

INSTRUCTIONS: Please process the above mentioned request.

APPROVED FOR RELEASED
DATE: 10-Jun-2009

PRIORITY HANDLING   FOIA REQUEST (b) (3)

SUBJECT: (Optional) Notification of a New Litigation		REQUEST NUMBER
Gilbert Roman v. NASA, NRO, CIA		F96-0018, F96-2158,
C.A. No. 1:97CV01164 (U.S.D.D.C.)		F97-0410, F97-0522,
		F97-0755, F97-0891 and

FROM:	EXTENSION	DATE SENT
		28 July 1997 P96-1518
		SUSPENSE DATE

TO: (Officer designation, room number, and building)	DATE		OFFICER'S INITIALS	COMMENTS (Number each comment to show from whom to whom. Draw a line across column after each comment.)
	RECEIVED	FORWARDED		

Comments:

Please be advised that this case is now the subject of a litigation for information on satellites owned by the CIA and for information on himself.

The current status of this case is a Closed Initial (ELI).

The attorney assigned to this case is [ ] A copy of the complaint is attached for your information.

DA: for information (P96-1518, F97-0755, F97-0522)

DO: for information (P96-1518)

DS&T: for information (F97-0755)

OGC: for information (A complete copy of the file has already been forwarded to you)

C.O.: [ ]

TO list:

1. DA/IRO
2.
3. DO/IRO
4.
5. DS&T/IRO
6.
7. OGC/LD via
8.
9.
10.
11.
12.

RETURN TO:

PRIORITY HANDLING   FOIA REQUEST

FORM 3749 (EF) OBSOLETE PREVIOUS EDITIONS
I-79

C05390983

(b) (3)

23 July 97

<u>Gilbert Roman v. NASA NRO CIA</u>

Civil Action no: <u>1:97CV01164 (U.S.D.D.C.)</u>
Judge Paul Friedman
Attorney: pro se

Litigation involves F96-0018, F96-2158,
F97-0410, F97-0522, F97-0755, F97-0891,
and P96-1518, info. on satellites owned
by CIA and info on self

Date Filed with OGC: 30 June 97
OGC Attorney:
OGC Paralegal:
RAB Case Officer: as of 10/27/97
Rec'd Date: 2 July 97

PLS. RETURN

Logging:

Please log in this new litigation as indicated: F96-0018, F96-
2158, F97-0410, F97-0522, F97-0755, F97-0891 (info on satellites
owned by CIA), P96-1518 (info on self).

Pre-litigation status is Closed Initial (ELI).

Thank you.

APPROVED FOR RELEASED
DATE: 10-Jun-2009

89

C05390984

(b) (3)

SECURE FACSIMILE TRANSMITTAL FORM

DATE: 3ᵗ July, 97

SENDING SECURE/FAX TELEPHONE NUMBER:
RECEIVING SECURE/FAX TELEPHONE NUMBER:
NUMBER OF PAGES (Including Transmittal Form and Coversheet if applicable)   2
FROM:
                    (Name / Office / Extension)
SUBJECT: Roman Litigation
TO: (ADDRESSEE / ORGANIZATION / OFFICE / EXTENSION)

1.
2.
3.
4.
5.
6.
7.
8.
9.
10.

What does he plan not to?)
respond to

SPECIAL INSTRUCTIONS: *This same in after the Summons/Complaint*
- I plan not to respond.

RELEASING OFFICIAL:
                    (PRINTED NAME)   (SIGNATURE)

RECEIVING STATION USE ONLY

Please receipt for material by entering time of receipt/signature and transmit back to sending station.

DATE / TIME: SIGNATURE:

FORM   4383A   (EF)
10-92   (CLASSIFICATION OF MATERIAL TRANSMITTED)

APPROVED FOR
RELEASE DATE:
10-Jun-2009

90

PRIVACY ACT REQUEST

SUBJECT: (Optional) RE: INFO ON SELF				REQUEST NUMBER	
ROMAN, GILBERT				P96-1518	

FROM:			EXTENSION	DATE SENT 5 August 1996	
IP&CRD/NSG/OIT				SUSPENSE DATE	

TO: (Officer designation, room number, and building)	DATE		OFFICER'S INITIALS	COMMENTS (Number each comment to show from whom to whom. Draw a line across column after each comment.)
	RECEIVED	FORWARDED		
1. DDA/IRO-Mr.Hatch 1236 Ames Bldg.		13/ A 9/6		Please process the attached Privacy request.
2. OPS oms				PLEASE PROCESS UNDER PA & FOIA
3.				SEARCH CUT OFF DATE: 30 July 96
4. RETURN TO: DDA/IRO-Mr.Hatch 1236 Ames Bldg.				FEE CATEGORY: No Fees
5.				PLS NOTE: CR: F96-8018
6. OMB				
7.				
8.				
9.				
10.				

ANOTHER FOIA REQUEST AND RUNAROUND

In this response, the NRO states that the CIA does not take FOIA request from intermediaries. This statement goes against the federal register (vol. 52, no. 235 on the rules and regulations). Please read.

institution of professional education and an institution of vocational education which operates a degree-granting, accredited program or programs of scholarly research in recognized fields of study. The criteria to be met to be included in this category, for the purposes of fee waivers, are not satisfied simply by showing that the request is for a library or other records repository. Such requests, like those of other requesters, will be analyzed to identify the particular person who will actually use the requested information in a scholarly or other analytic work and then disseminate it to the general public.

(p) "Non-commercial scientific institution" refers to an institution in the United States that is not operated on a "commercial" basis as that term is referenced in paragraph (n) of this section and which is operated solely for the purpose of conducting natural life or physical sciences research the results of which are not intended to promote any particular product or industry.

(q) "Representatives of the news media" refers to any person actively gathering news for a United States entity that is organized and operated to publish or broadcast news in the United States to the general public. The term "news" means information that is about current events or that would be of current interest to the general public. Examples of news media entities include television or radio stations broadcasting to the public at large and publishers of printed periodicals (but only in those instances when they qualify as disseminators of "news") who make their products available for purchase or subscription by the general public and whose products are, in fact, received by a significant element of the general public. These examples are not intended to be all-inclusive. Moreover, as traditional methods of news delivery evolve (e.g., electronic dissemination of newspapers through telecommunications services), such alternative media would be included in this category. In the case of "freelance" journalists, they may be regarded as working for a news organization if they can demonstrate a solid basis for expecting publication through that organization, even though not actually employed by it. A publication contract would be the clearest proof, but the requester's past publication record may also be relevant evidence of the requester's status.

§ 1900.5   Organization; requests and submittals.

The headquarters of the Central Intelligence Agency is located in Fairfax

County, VA. Functions are channeled and determined by regular chain-of-command procedures. Except as provided by this regulation, there are no formal or informal procedural requirements regarding public access to Agency records. Requests and other submittals should be addressed to: Information and Privacy Coordinator, Central Intelligence Agency, Washington, DC 20505.

Requesting Records

§ 1900.11   Freedom of Information Act and Executive Order 12356 communications; requirements as to form.

(a) Any communication to the CIA or to the Director of Central Intelligence under the Freedom of Information Act or Executive Order 12356 should be addressed to: Information and Privacy Coordinator, Central Intelligence Agency, Washington, D.C. 20505. This address should appear on the envelope or other folder or package in which the communication is transmitted. It should also be included as the addressee of the letter or other communication or be clearly set forth in the text of the communication.

(b) Any request for records under the Freedom of Information Act (§ 1900.35), expression of interest in requesting records (§ 1900.35) or request for declassification of records under Executive Order 12356 (§ 1900.35) shall be in writing and shall be addressed as prescribed by § 1900.11(a). The Coordinator may, but need not, waive the requirements as to address.

(c) The request or expression of interest shall reasonably describe the records of interest and, in the case of mandatory declassification review, requests shall identify the documents(s) with specificity such as by National Archives and Records Administration (NARA) Document Accession Number or other applicable, unique document identifying number.

(d) Any request or communications to an agency other than the Central Intelligence Agency which concern documents, records or information originated by the CIA and referred to the CIA, shall be considered a Freedom of Information request to the CIA for that referred document as of date of receipt by the CIA of the referral, and shall be processed pursuant to regulations.

§ 1900.21   Identification of persons requesting information under the provisions of Executive Order 12356.

Pursuant to section 3.4(a)(1) of Executive Order 12356, a mandatory declassification review request can be made only by a United States citizen or

permanent resident alien, a federal agency or a State or local government. This Agency shall require sufficient identifying information from the requester to authenticate the requester's qualifications.

§ 1900.23   Pre-request option: Estimates of charges.

(a) In order to avoid being faced with unanticipated sizeable charges, interested persons and entities may defer the submission of requests for records and first submit a written request, in accordance with the procedures prescribed by § 1900.11 for an estimate of charges likely to be incurred if the records are requested.

(b) Notice is hereby given that a requester may be liable for the payment of search charges, in accordance with the fee schedule and provisions of § 1900.25, even if search for requested records locates no such records and even if some or all of requested records which are located are denied the requester under one or more exemptions of the Freedom of Information Act or Executive Order 12356.

§ 1900.25   Fees for records services.

(a) Search, review, and duplication fees will be charged in accordance with the schedule set forth in paragraph (c) of this section for services rendered in responding to requests for Agency records under this part. To the extent possible, the most efficient and least costly methods will be used to comply with requests for documents made under the FOIA. Records will be furnished without charge or at a reduced rate whenever the Coordinator determines that a waiver or reduction is in the public interest because it is likely to contribute significantly to public understanding of the operations or activities of the United States government and is not primarily in the commerical interest of the requester. The Coordinator shall consider the following factors in making his determination:

(1) Whether the subject of the requested records concerns the operations or activities of the United States government; and, if so.

(2) Whether the disclosure of the requested documents is likely to contribute to an understanding of United States government operations or activities; and, if so,

(3) Whether the disclosure of the requested documents will contribute to public understanding of United States government operations or activities; and, if so,

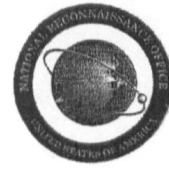

NATIONAL RECONNAISSANCE OFFICE
14675 Lee Road
Chantilly, VA 20151-1715

Information Access and Release Center   11 March 1997
(703) 808-5029

Mr. Gilbert Roman

Case Number F97-0002

Dear Mr. Roman:

The Information Access and Release Center of the National Reconnaissance Office has received a response (attached) from the Central Intelligence Agency (CIA) with regard to our referral of you 19 December 1996 Freedom of Information Act (FOIA) request.

It is the CIA's policy not to accept FOIA requests from intermediaries, so they have returned your request to us.

Since you are specifically requesting information about the CIA, we recommend that you contact them directly. You can address your request to:

> Information and Privacy Coordinator
> Central Intelligence Agency
> Washington, DC 20505

Sincerely,

BARBARA E. FREIMANN
Chief, Information Access
and Release Center

Attachment

ANOTHER NSA FOIA CASE NO. 09-2947

In this case, I asked for information on FMRI technology—the date it was put into service and the report on the first person it was used successfully. The NSA refused to make searches, claiming it does not fall into their purview. I made an appeal, which was never answered. Proof of service is in the following papers (PR).

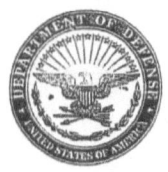

NATIONAL SECURITY AGENCY
CENTRAL SECURITY SERVICE

FORT GEORGE G. MEADE, MARYLAND 20755-6000

FOIA Case: 58310
1 April 2009

Mr. Gilbert Roman
95-25 77th Street
Ozone Park, NY 11416

Dear Mr. Roman:

This responds to your Freedom of Information Act (FOIA) request of 6 March 2009, which was received by this office on 11 March 2009, for information on functional magnetic resonance imaging, the date it was put into service, and the first successful report on the first person it was used on successfully.

For purposes of this request and based on the information you provided in your letter, you are considered an "all other" requester. As such, you are allowed 2 hours of search and the duplication of 100 pages at no cost. There are no assessable fees for this request.

The National Security Agency/Central Security Service (NSA/CSS) is the nation's cryptologic organization, and we have a twofold mission. Our Information Assurance mission is to provide solutions, products, and services to protect U.S. information infrastructures critical to national security interests. In response to requirements set at the highest levels of government, our Signals intelligence mission is to collect, process, and disseminate intelligence information from foreign signals for national foreign intelligence and counterintelligence purposes and to support military operations. Therefore, the information you request does not fall within the purview of this Agency, and a search for records responsive to your request would not be productive.

The fact that we have determined the subject of your request does not fall within the purview of this Agency may be considered by you as an adverse determination. You are hereby advised of this Agency's appeal procedures. Any person notified of an adverse determination may file an appeal to the NSA/CSS Freedom of Information Act Appeal Authority. The appeal must be postmarked no later than 60 calendar days after the date of the initial denial letter. The appeal shall be in writing addressed to the NSA/CSS FOIA Appeal Authority (DJP4), National Security Agency, 9800 Savage Road STE 6248, Fort George G. Meade, MD 20755-6248. To aid in processing the appeal, it should reference the adverse determination and explain in sufficient detail and particularity the grounds upon which you believe a search is warranted. The NSA/CSS FOIA Appeal Authority will endeavor to respond to the appeal within 20 working days after receipt, absent unusual circumstances.

We have enclosed a fact sheet describing NSA/CSS's mission, which we hope you will find useful and informative.

Sincerely,

PAMELA N. PHILLIPS
Acting Initial Denial Authority

Gilbert Roman
95-25 77th st
Ozone Pk., NY 11416

Re: FOIA CASE # 58310

   This is an appeal of your denial letter dated April 1, 2009. This appeal is made under the Freedom of Information Act and/or privacy Act of 1974. I request the release of all requested information. I am a US citizen and as such you should guide me to which agency has these records. Attached you shall find copies of my request and your denial.

   Thank You.

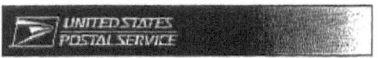

Track/Confirm - Intranet Item Inquiry
Item Number: 7008 1140 0000 9512 4068

The item(s) you queried are summarized below. If you would like to request a delivery record check the box in the "Select" column to the right of the item (if available). Learn more about Restore.

Detail	Item	Origin	Destination	Firm	Recipient	Event/Image Info	Date	Time	Sele
Archived	70081140000095124068		20755		EVERD	DELIVERED	4/10/2009	12:51	☐

Request Delivery Record for Selected Items

Enter Request Type and Item Number:

Quick Search ◉   Extensive Search ○

Explanation of Quick and Extensive Searches

Submit

Version 1.0

Inquire on multiple items.

Go to the Product Tracking System Home Page.

(NSA) They never answered my appeal

99

Central Intelligence Agency

Washington, D.C. 20505

Other papers of support:

JUN 10 , 1999

Mr. Gilbert Roman

Reference: F-1999-00952

Dear Mr. Roman:

This is in response to your 21 April 1999 Freedom of Information Act (FOIA) request for records you describe as follows:

[1] "I request copies of the forms used to process all of my FOIA and/or PA request to your agency and be certain to include all computer log-sheet time used to search for my request."

[2] "I request satellite surveillance records of a person being monitored in the Woodbridge/Middlesex County, NJ area in 1987-1991; Brooklyn, NY area in 1991-1995; Ogdensburg, NY area 1995-1997.

We have assigned your request the reference number above for identification purposes. Please refer to it in any future correspondence.

With regard to item 1 only—copies of forms used to process your FOIA requests—we have accepted your request; it will be processed in accordance with the FOIA, 5 U.S.C. § 552, as amended, and the CIA Information Act, 50 U.S.C. § 431. Our search will be for documents in existence as of and through the date of this acceptance letter.

Because we believe that fees would be minimal, and as an act of administrative discretion, we have determined that no fees will be charged for this request.

The heavy volume of FOIA requests received by the Agency has created delays in processing. Since we cannot respond within the 20 working days stipulated by the Act, you have the right to consider this as a denial and may appeal to the Agency Release Panel. It would seem more reasonable, however, to have us continue processing your request and respond as soon as we can. You can appeal any denial of records at that time. Unless we hear from you otherwise, we will assume that you agree, and we will proceed on this basis.

With regard to item 2—satellite records—the CIA can neither confirm nor deny the existence or nonexistence of records responsive to your request. Such information—unless it has been official acknowledged—would be classified for reasons of national security under Executive Order 12958. The fact of the existence or nonexistence of such records would also relate directly to information concerning intelligence sources and methods. The Director of Central Intelligence has the responsibility and authority to protect such information from unauthorized disclosure in accordance with Subsection 103(c)(6) of the National Security Act of 1947 and Section 6 of the CIA Act of 1949. Therefore, your request is denied under FOIA exemptions (b)(1) and (b)(3); an explanation of these exemptions is enclosed.

The CIA official responsible for this determination is Lee S. Strickland, Information and Privacy Coordinator. By this action we are neither confirming nor denying the existence or nonexistence of such records. You may appeal this decision by addressing your appeal to the Agency Release Panel, in my care, within 45 days from the date of our final response to this request.

We will contact you again when we have completed processing item 1 of your request.

Sincerely,

Lee S. Strickland
Information and Privacy Coordinator

Enclosure

Mr. Gilbert Roman

Reference: F96-2158

Dear Mr. Roman:

This is in response to your letter of 7 December 1996 to John Deutch, Director of Central Intelligence, wherein you requested the following information:

"1) The names of all satellites in orbit as of 1986 until present date under the control of the Central intelligence agency [sic]"

"2) The built in [sic] capabilities"

"3) The copy to develop each one"

"4) The names of all scientist and medical doctors assigned to the development of these satellites and their biographic backgrounds"

"5) The cost of each built in [sic] capability"

"6) Which one reads the thoughts of the person in is focused on"

Your letter was forwarded to the office of the Information and Privacy Coordinator for response to you. For identification purposes we have assigned your request the number referenced above.

Your request, given its lack of specificity, is unsearchable in our records systems and therefore, cannot be processed. More specifically, the FOIA provides for public access to "reasonably described" records. This means that documents must be described sufficiently to enable to professional employee familiar with the subject to locate the document without an unreasonable amount of effort. Commonly this equates to a requirement that the documents must be locatable through the indexing to our various records. In sum, the FOIA does not require federal agencies to perform research or to conduct unreasonable searches through a body of material to see if any of it is related to a particular request.

We regret we cannot be of assistance to you.

Sincerely,

Lee S. Strickland
Information and Privacy Coordinator

102

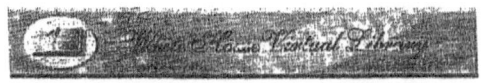

White House Press Release

RELEASE OF IMAGERY ACQUIRED BY SPACE-BASED NATIONAL INTELLIGENCE RECONNAISSANCE SYSTEMS

THE WHITE HOUSE

Office of the Press Secretary

For Immediate Release   February 24, 1995

EXECUTIVE ORDER
#12951
- - - - - - -

RELEASE OF IMAGERY ACQUIRED BY SPACE-BASED
NATIONAL INTELLIGENCE RECONNAISSANCE SYSTEMS

By the authority vested in me as President by the Constitution and the laws of the United States of America and in order to release certain scientifically or environmentally useful imagery acquired by space-based national intelligence reconnaissance systems, consistent with the national security, it is hereby ordered as follows:

Section 1. Public Release of Historical Intelligence Imagery. Imagery acquired by the space-based national intelligence reconnaissance systems known as the Corona, Argon, and Lanyard missions shall, within 18 months of the date of this order, be declassified and transferred to the National Archives and Records Administration with a copy sent to the United States Geological Survey of the Department of the Interior consistent with procedures approved by the Director of Central Intelligence and the Archivist of the United States. Upon transfer, such imagery shall be deemed declassified and shall be made available to the public.

Sec. 2. Review for Future Public Release of Intelligence Imagery. (a) All information that meets the criteria in section 2(b) of this order shall be kept secret in the interests of national defense and foreign policy until deemed otherwise by the Director of Central Intelligence. In consultation with the Secretaries of State and Defense, the Director of Central Intelligence shall establish a comprehensive program for the periodic review of imagery from systems other than the Corona, Argon, and Lanyard missions, with the objective of making available to the public as much imagery as possible consistent

E-①

CONCLUSION

We, the people, must be certain that this technology is used properly. Author James Bamford once stated that the NSA had bin Laden's cell number, his relay house in Yemen under surveillance (where bin Laden would call in orders), and at least two of the September 11 hijackers under surveillance. Then why did the September 11 attack happen? Yes, FMRI technology will be used in the medical field. It is because of the possible misuse that strict guidelines must be placed on it.

I BELIEVE THAT FMRI TECHNOLOGY IS BUILT INTO SATELLITES!

I BELIEVE THAT FMRI TECHNOLOGY IS IN MOBILE UNITS!

I BELIEVE THAT FMRI TECHNOLOGY IS IN STATIONARY UNITS!

I BELIEVE THAT FMRI TECHNOLOGY COULD BE TARGETED THROUGH CAMERAS!

I BELIEVE THAT FMRI TECHNOLOGY COULD TARGET INDIVIDUALS WITH BINOCULARS!

www.ingramcontent.com/pod-product-compliance
Lightning Source LLC
Chambersburg PA
CBHW022019170526
45157CB00003B/1283